BEAUTY
&
CANCER

BEAUTY
&
CANCER

Looking and Feeling Your Best

Diane Doan Noyes *written by* Peggy Mellody R.N.

Taylor Publishing Company
Dallas, Texas

Published by Taylor Publishing Company
1550 West Mockingbird Lane
Dallas, Texas 75235

Design: Paula Bingham Goldstein

Art Direction: Bill Brown

Illustrations: Ann Noyes

Library of Congress Cataloging-in-Publication Data

Noyes, Diane Doan.
    Beauty & Cancer : a woman's guide to looking great while
experiencing the side effects of cancer therapy / Diane Doan Noyes;
written by Peggy Mellody ; [illustrations, Ann Noyes].
            p.   cm.
    Originally published: Los Angeles : AC Press, 1988.
    Includes bibliographical references (p.145) and index.
    ISBN 0-87833-809-8 $12.95
    1. Women--Health and hygiene.   2. Cancer--Treatment--
Complications and sequelae.   3. Beauty, Personal.   4. Cancer--Patients
--Rehabilitation.   I. Mellody, Peggy.   II. Title.   III. Title: Beauty
and cancer.
[RC281.W65N69   1992]
646.7'042'0877--dc20   92-14254
                                                                       CIP

Printed in the United States of America

10   9   8   7   6   5   4   3

In memory of Laura Friedman.

She filled our hearts and touched our lives with her youth, courage, and enthusiasm.

TABLE OF
CONTENTS

A Patient Observed:

When you look good on the outside, you'll feel good on the inside, and feeling good about yourself is an important step in coping with cancer.

CHANGES, CHOICES, AND CHALLENGES

PREFACE

On May 6, 1986 I was diagnosed with ovarian cancer. It was as if someone had placed a brick wall in front of me. Immediately, I was confronted with the numerous available options which might help rid all the cancerous cells from my body. Once my cancer had been surgically removed, unless it was aggressively treated with what my doctor referred to as "industrial strength" chemotherapy, it still had a 95% chance of returning within three months. I didn't really know anyone who had received chemotherapy, so I was unaware of what to expect during the next year. My physician and nurses explained the physical changes that can occur with chemotherapy, but I was unprepared for the psychological impact of these side effects.

Two weeks after my first chemotherapy treatment my hair began to fall out. Within four weeks I experienced total hair loss -- scalp hair, eyebrows, and eyelashes. Along with suffering from nausea and fatigue, I felt like my life was suddenly put on hold until the whole ordeal was over. Fortunately for me, my family and friends decided they were not going to allow me to feel sorry for myself. Realizing my financial obligations, my job, and my family's dependency on me I had to continue to maintain a normal daily existence. I decided that I was going to be a cancer survivor. I believed that if I could look good, I'd feel better.

I found, however, when it came to finding information, organized programs, or assistance on how to cope with the physical side effects of cancer treatments, there was little valuable help. I discovered stores are stocked only for seasonal shoppers and their sales staffs had little knowledge of how the products could adversely affect or help the woman with cancer. Along with the devastating feeling of being totally unattractive, I was forced to recognize the fact that there was nothing available to assist me.

Faced with this dilemma I began experimenting, by trial and error, with fabric and makeup to counteract the physical side effects I was experiencing. One of the many mistakes I made along the way was buying a wig before my hair fell out, so by the time I needed it, the wig didn't fit.

I found using scarves as headwraps were the best solution while my hair was growing back. My stepmother taught me how to tie and make headwraps that were easy and appropriate for all occasions. In addition to making my own fashion statement, my ego and self esteem were constantly getting a boost from all the compliments I received. In fact, many of my clients, business associates, and friends didn't even realize I did not have hair. I'm convinced that pampering myself and taking the extra time to deal with my beauty needs improved my attitude to the point where I was better able to tolerate the chemotherapy and as a result recovered quicker.

I learned a lot about myself and realized that even in this age of information few tools are available to help women with cancer improve their physical appearance and body image. While I was going through my chemotherapy treatments, I met a lot of women with different cancers and a variety of problems related specifically to their disease and treatment. They, like I, felt isolated from society because of the lack of resources available to teach us how to combat these physical symptoms. Although I was able to develop my own beauty strategy, it was a long and often frustrating process. I still had a lot to learn about my own side effects, but as my hair and skin came back to normal, I didn't want other women to go through the same experience. With the encouragement of my oncologist, I decided that a book would be the best initial source of information for not only women with cancer, but for health and beauty professionals as well.

In order to meet the needs of the majority of women with cancer, I sought out the experience of a cancer professional. Peggy Mellody's experience as an oncology nurse specialist, author, and health care consultant made us the perfect team.

In 1988, the first edition of *Beauty & Cancer* was published. Peggy and I knew that the key to the book's success would be making sure that the people who needed the information (the person with cancer) would know the information was there. To achieve this goal, the book was immediately introduced to the oncology community, particularly to the nurses who are the key to providing patient education and product referrals. They quickly embraced the book as a valuable resource and immediately began to share the information in the book with their patients.

Individuals with cancer are very generous with others in similar situations by sharing information about their disease. As a result, news of *Beauty & Cancer* was quickly exchanged between them. In fact, many of Peggy's patients, not realizing who she was, would bring her copies of *Beauty & Cancer* and say, "You should know about this book." By 1989, due mainly to the networking of nurses and patients, *Beauty & Cancer* had been sold in over 15 countries, demonstrating the fact that the information in the book had no international boundaries.

Recognizing the importance of personal appearance and body image in the recovery process of women, men, and children with cancer, we developed a consulting firm called "Appearance Concepts." Appearance Concepts provides information on managing the appearance side effects of cancer therapies, new product development, merchandising to the customer with cancer, and survivorship issues. The information is provided through seminars to health care professionals, to individuals of all ages with cancer, to their families, and to beauty and fashion professionals.

During the last four years, Peggy and I have been witness to a change in the services offered by the cancer care community; oncology professionals are learning creative approaches to symptom management, which includes appearance; the fashion/cosmetic industry is responding to their customer's special needs by creating or improving products; appearance consultants specializing in the needs of the person with cancer are available nationwide; and many cancer centers are now providing on-site image programs.

The future is brighter for all women with cancer. Together Peggy and I have developed a beauty program that we hope will improve your appearance and body image plus give you the strength and courage to complete your cancer treatments and join the ranks of cancer survivors.

Diane

ACKNOWLEDGEMENTS

The success of this project is due to the support of many special people. The encouragement from my family— Mom, Peter, Joshua, Paul, Dad, Betty, and Debbie— since the time I was diagnosed has been a great source of love, strength, and courage.

I am especially thankful to Dr. Joanna Cain, my oncologist, whose decision for aggressive treatment enabled me to be here today, and who was always there to answer my questions and help ease my fears.

Last, a sincere appreciation to my neighbors, friends, family, and co-workers for all their moral support and prayers.

D.D.N.

ACKNOWLEDGEMENTS

It is through the help of many people and educational resources that this book's contents came to be. I am especially grateful to all the organizations and people who contributed their experience, expertise, and time during the development of this book—Chris Saul; Margaret Murray, R.D.; Gerrie Pickney; Lynn Schokley; Paula Adams; Linda Secher; Peggy Knight; The American Cancer Society; The National Institute of Health; and The United Ostomy Association.

I deeply appreciate the interest, encouragement, and assistance from my husband, family, and friends from the beginning to end of this project.

Finally, a special thanks to the Oncology Nursing Society; Bernie Friedman; Craig and Flori Roberts, Dermablend; Joanna Cain, M.D., University of Washington Medical Center; Barbara Gauthier; Sharon Jamison, Adria Laboratories; Gary S. Lazar, M.D., University of California Los Angeles; and Linda Rose, Darci Dillard, and Joan Williams for their constant interest and support.

P.M.

1
ABOUT THIS BOOK

E very year nearly 500,000 American women are diagnosed and treated for some form of cancer. Contrary to the stereotype of the hospitalized patient, a large percentage of these women are receiving chemotherapy and radiation as an out-patient while continuing their careers, going to school, and caring for their families. Unfortunately, the side effects of these treatments can make women feel too frightened and embarrassed to return to the work place or feel a part of society. In fact, women who do remain on the job may feel unable to reach their potential and may be discriminated against for not matching the company's "image". Women with cancer may suffer more from society's reaction to them than they do from their disease.

Women with cancer may suffer more from society's reaction to them than they do from their disease.

Traditionally the emotional and physical side effects of cancer treatments have been something women were expected to grin and bear. The prevailing attitude has been that being "happy to be alive" is more important than how a woman looks, and how her appearance affects the quality of her life. Women have been expected to just make do with no hair, alterations in skin color, loss of facial features, and ill-fitting clothes. Until now -- *Beauty & Cancer* is designed to help overcome some of the fear, intimidation, and isolation women feel during and after cancer therapies, by improving their control of their appearance and their comfort. This book provides the information and resources for looking great, while experiencing the side effects of chemotherapy, radiation, and surgery.

This is a handbook for self indulgence. Historically, women have felt that they should be all things to all people at the same time. To maintain the "super-woman" role it has been necessary to juggle family responsibilities, career obligations, and health concerns, leaving little time for herself. If you have never taken the time to pamper yourself, do it now. Cancer treatments often make people feel helpless, dependent, and lacking in self worth. If you have recently been diagnosed with cancer you may be asking, "Why me?" You may be feeling angry at the world, your family, and/or your disease, or feeling depressed because your life has suddenly been disrupted. All of these feelings are normal and are experienced in varying degrees by most people in the same situation. Instead of focusing on what has happened to you, try directing your energy and thoughts towards what you can and will do for yourself. By doing things for yourself you will feel that you are regaining some control of your life, and feel good about yourself in the process. In fact, positive attitudes and high self esteem play a major role in the healing process.

This book is not a textbook on the differences between cancers, the causes of cancer, or the treatments for cancer. Cancer therapies are sophisticated and very individualized. What is good for you may not be for someone else, and visa versa. Your own oncologist is the best source of information regarding your disease and its treatments. We are not recommending one form of therapy over another, but recognize that there are many facets of the treatment plan for cancer. Therefore, the information presented in this book should be used in conjunction with the cancer therapies outlined for you by your doctor.

The major forms of cancer treatments are chemotherapy, radiation, and surgery. Depending upon the disease being treated, one or more of these therapies may be used.

CHEMOTHERAPY

Chemotherapy is the use of "anti-cancer" or "anti-tumor" drugs to kill and control cancer cells' development. These drugs can be given by mouth (orally), injected under the skin (subcutaneously), injected into a muscle (intramuscularly), injected into a vein (intravenously), or injected into the abdomen (intraperitoneal). Chemotherapeutic drugs may be given alone, in combination with other drugs, and in addition to radiation or surgery (adjuvant chemotherapy).

Cancer cells rapidly reproduce and grow in an uncontrolled manner. Chemotherapy suppresses the cancer cells' growth by interfering with their ability to divide. Unfortunately, these drugs also affect normal cells that naturally reproduce quickly (i.e., bone marrow, lining of the mouth and gut, and hair follicles). These toxic effects to normal cells can cause a host of unpleasant side effects. Bone marrow manufactures three types of blood cells, each with their own function: red blood cells (erythrocytes) carry oxygen to the body's tissues, platelets (thrombocytes) help prevent bleeding by clotting the blood, and white blood cells (leukocytes) provide the body with its main line of defense against infection. When the bone marrow is not functioning properly, fatigue, bleeding gums or easy bruising, and increased risk of infections are common. Be aware of

Be aware of your blood counts and the precautions you should take if they are low.

your blood counts and the precautions you should take if they are low. For example, if your white cell count or platelet count is decreased, try to prevent potential sources of infections and bleeding such as cuts and scratches in the skin. Additionally, you may need to be especially careful about what beauty products and techniques you use on your skin.

Nausea and vomiting, mouth sores, indigestion, and digestive problems are frequent results of chemotherapy's effect on the lining of the mouth, stomach and intestines.

Hair loss may be chemotherapy's most devastating side effect for women and usually occurs approximately two to three weeks after the initiation of therapy. The loss of hair may start as a gradual thinning or suddenly come out in clumps; however, there is no way to accurately predict how each individual will react to the drugs they will be receiving. In addition to the scalp hair, eyebrows, eyelashes, pubic hair, and other body hair may also be lost, but the most common area of hair loss is the scalp. Fortunately, most of these side effects are temporary, and go away as the normal cells recover. In fact, in many cases the hair grows back looking healthier and more beautiful than before chemotherapy. Complete or partial hair loss is determined by the use of certain chemotherapy agents and is often related to the total dose received. Common offenders of complete hair loss include: cyclophosphomide (Cytoxan®), daunorubicin, and doxorubicin (Adriamycin®), ifosfamide (Ifex®). Further, many other chemotherapy agents and medications have the potential for causing complete or partial hair loss, especially when combination drug therapy is used. As the hair bulb shrinks from exposure to toxic drugs, hair is lost.

Recently a technique called scalp hypothermia has been developed which helps protect against hair loss by decreasing the scalp's temperature near the hair bulb. An "ice turban" or "chemo cap" is worn for 10 to 15 minutes before and after receiving chemotherapy. This technique is considered by some physicians and insurance companies as experimental and only may be beneficial in conjunction with specific types and doses of chemotherapy, and appropriate only for certain cancers. Be sure to consult your physician about this procedure, since it can be detrimental when used with specific cancers, especially those involving the bone marrow (i.e., leukemia) and when tumor cells are present in the scalp. The F.D.A. has placed restrictions on the purchase and use of hypothermia caps.

In general, hair regrowth occurs about three weeks after the completion of chemotherapy, but in some cases hair will grow back in between cycles of chemotherapy, and then usually falls out again. Scalp hair grows at an average rate of 1/2 inch per month.

RADIATION

Radiation therapy is used to kill cancer cells in a discrete location. Radiation is used as the main treatment for some forms of cancer, and used in conjunction with chemotherapy and surgery for other cancers. It is also an effective treatment to relieve some of the symptoms of cancer such as pain (palliative radiation therapy).

There are several forms of radiation therapy. It can be administered from outside the body via special "megavoltage" x-ray machines whose radiation

7

penetrates deep inside the body, avoiding healthy tissue as much as possible. Or it can be administered internally, with a radioactive implant that is placed in the body next to or directly into the tumor. Radiation, like chemotherapy, is toxic to normal cells, but radiation's main side effects are specific to the area treated, not generalized. Possible side effects of radiation include fatigue, dry skin, changes in the fingernails' color and appearance, nausea and vomiting, changes in taste perception, changes in skin color, skin burns, and hair loss.

Radiation therapy affects hair only in the treatment area. The type and total dose of radiation administered will determine whether the hair loss will be permanent or temporary. Also, radiation therapy may retard hair growth and regrowth may begin several months after the last treatment. Be sure to discuss hair loss as well as potential side effects with your radiation oncologist.

SURGERY

Beauty is a combination of skin care, makeup, hair, diet and exercise, and positive attitudes.

Surgery is used to remove the cancerous tumor, any tissues affected by the cancer cells, and tissue that might have yet undetected cancer cells. Surgery's main side effect is often psychological, making women feel disfigured or robbed of their femininity due to the removal of tissue (i.e., breast or uterus), and/or the addition of a prosthesis or external tubes and bags (i.e., breast implant, colostomy bag).

Each chapter of this book provides the tools for creating a new-looking you, maybe even a better-looking you. Personal beauty comes from the interest you take in yourself. Beauty is a combination of skin care, makeup,

8

hair, diet and exercise, and positive attitudes. It requires an ongoing commitment, ideally beginning before you start your cancer therapy and then continuing beyond your treatment. Clothes, makeup, hairstyles, and headwraps that make you look good are an important bridge to the healthy world.

The first step to maintaining control is to think of yourself as a woman, not as a patient. The word "patient" often has negative connotations and can place many people in a dependent role. By thinking of your treatments as an inconvenience or interruption in your life, and not the only part of your life, you'll be sending a message that says you haven't given up and are willing to face the challenges ahead of you. For example, if you are hospitalized, wear your own nightgowns to avoid looking institutionalized. Let your personality shine through by using makeup and headwraps. Even if you only wear lip gloss and a hint of blush you'll look and feel better.

Become an active participant in the fight for your recovery.

If you are going to a clinic or your doctor's office for your treatments, take the time to wear clothes, makeup, and headpieces that make your own individualized fashion statement. The staff and other patients will take notice and the compliments will begin to pour in. Positive attitudes can be infectious. The confidence you exhibit will spread to the medical staff caring for you and to the other women with cancer waiting for their treatments. You will become a role model for other women with cancer. Fear breeds fear. The lack of fear you demonstrate may give others some of the courage and positive self image you possess.

Next, become an active participant in the fight for your recovery, so that your physicians and nurses don't have

9

to carry the battle alone. This may be your first experience with being sick and the busy routines of doctor offices, clinics, and hospitals, so you may be feeling a bit intimidated and unsure of what is considered acceptable behavior by you. Throughout this process you may be feeling rushed into deciding from a variety of options regarding the treatment of your disease. You may feel that you are losing control and that others are making decisions for you. Many individuals slip into the dependent and often vulnerable role of a patient, laying back and verbally or non-verbally saying, "Do what you will."

Knowledge is a powerful tool.

To stop the cycle, you must tell yourself that you are in control and will be involved in the decision making process of your care. Remember, your health care is a shared responsibility between you and the health care team. Knowledge is a powerful tool. Commonly, people leave their physician feeling frustrated and thinking information is being withheld or their questions haven't been answered. If you have questions, ask them! There is no such thing as a dumb question. Write down your questions prior to seeing your doctor. If you're hospitalized, keep a pad and pencil near your bed to write down questions as you think of them. Simply ask your physician to sit down for a few minutes so you can review your questions and concerns with him/her. Let your doctor know how much information you want and how often—daily, weekly, or monthly.

You have the right, and your physician has the obligation, to inform you of the risks and benefits of the treatments being offered you and other forms of treatments available. For surgery, not only do the risks and benefits need to be reviewed, but a description of

the surgical procedure and exactly what will be removed
and/or placed (i.e., prosthesis) must be provided. You
will be asked to sign a surgical consent; sign it only
after the procedure has been explained to you.

Develop a strategy for circumventing each potential
problem (i.e., hair loss) before it arrives. If possible,
before starting chemotherapy and radiation complete the
following checklist.

- See your dentist for a complete checkup. Tell your
  dentist that you have been diagnosed with cancer and
  will be starting chemotherapy and/or radiation soon.
  Have your teeth cleaned and your mouth and teeth
  inspected for potential sources of infections (i.e.,
  cavities). People who have good dental hygiene
  before starting chemotherapy are decreasing their
  risk of developing infections during and following
  chemotherapy.

- Discuss with your dentist, physician, or nurse
  guidelines for daily oral care during therapy, as well
  as any restrictions regarding having dental work done
  during this time.

- Discuss strategies for preventing potential side
  effects such as hair loss.

- Cut your hair short before starting chemotherapy.
  Hair loss related to chemotherapy tends to fall out in
  clumps, making women with long hair more
  uncomfortable than those with short hair.

- Cut and label pieces of hair form the top of your
  head, the side, and in the back at the nape of the neck
  to aid in selecting a natural appearing wig.

- Buy new nightgowns, slippers, and robes. Front opening gowns are best when you're in the hospital.

- Buy cotton scarves for headwraps.

- Purchase or make a flannel sleeping cap. A large amount of heat leaves through the top of your head. If your hair falls out, you may need a cap to substitute as insulation.

- Buy makeup—blush, eyebrow pencils, lipstick, foundation, and powder—and disposable makeup applicators for use when you are at risk of infection.

- Be familiar with your blood cell counts and the precautions you should take if one or more of them are low.

- Develop a resource list which includes the names and phone numbers of community resources you will need to tap, such as the American Cancer Society, wig salons, and specialty stores.

- Develop a personal beauty worksheet that includes brands and colors of makeup and skin care products, your eye color, hair color, and skin tone. Attach a color picture of yourself before you started chemotherapy and radiation.

- Review your insurance policy regarding coverage for prosthetics (hair or breast).

We hope the information contained in these chapters will help you look great and feel good about your personal appearance and body image while modern medicine works to heal you on the inside.

2
HAIR ALTERNATIVES

H air throughout the centuries has had powerful influences on individuals and society. It has meant strength, power, politics, wealth, and beauty. Its styling, color, and length can make social statements as well as portray an individual's personality and feelings. The loss of hair (alopecia), partial or complete, is one of the most common side effects of chemotherapy and radiation, and is considered by the majority of women as the most physically and emotionally devastating result of cancer therapy. Many women feel that the loss of hair is as difficult to deal with as the diagnosis of cancer. Unfortunately, health-care professionals are usually so busy attending to other needs that they lack the time to provide hair alternatives. Often nurses and physicians only offer the reassurance that it will grow back, but not the tools to cope and make adjustments with during the time you are without hair.

Women with cancer are not the only ones to experience hair loss. A condition called Alopecia Areata results in the loss of hair on the scalp and elsewhere. Although the exact cause of this condition is unknown, it is thought to be an autoimmune process in which the body's immune system reacts against its hair follicles (the structures which make hair grow) causing hair to be shed. It is not uncommon for women with Alopecia Areata to lose all their body hair instead of just scalp and facial hair, and in many cases the loss is permanent.

In the past, the only thing available for women without a full head of hair were cheap, ill-fitting hair pieces sold in department stores by clerks who had little or no training in wigs -- styling, care, or selection -- especially for the woman with total hair loss of the scalp. Today, wigs are available that look and feel as natural as your own hair. In fact, many of these wigs are easier to care for than your original hair.

WIG SELECTION

Choosing the right wig (hair prosthesis) can be a difficult decision. During a time of stress there are many people available to capitalize on your vulnerability and sell you a wig that is not suitable for you. The best wig for you will be one that:

- Appears natural looking.

- Feels comfortable and fits well.

- Fits your budget.

When you go to purchase a wig be sure to ask three questions:

1. What kind of hair is the wig made of?

2. How is the wig made?

3. How do you attach the wig to the scalp?

It is important to go to a store that offers privacy and individual attention, such as a shop specializing in wigs whose sales staff has experience dealing with women with cancer or traumatic hair loss. No woman without hair will feel comfortable trying on a hair prosthesis in the middle of a busy department store. When you go to purchase a wig be sure to ask three questions:

1. What kind of hair is the wig made of?

Wigs are made out of either a synthetic fiber, human hair, or a combination of these two.

2. How is the wig made?

Wigs are constructed in two major ways—machine-made and hand-tied (pre-custom and full-custom). Machine-made wigs are often thought of as being made for people with hair, but this is not always the case. In fact, many women find these wigs to be comfortable, as well as economical. These ready-made wigs are chosen by hair style, hair color, and head size (ranging from petite to large). Since all heads don't come in uniform sizes, machine-made wigs can be easily altered for a near-custom fit. The bases of machine-made wigs are composed of cotton wefts to which the hair, usually synthetic, is sewn. If you are experiencing total hair loss, select a wig that has the wefts close together.

Pre-custom, hand-tied wigs are made for individuals experiencing partial or total hair loss. The hair is hand-knotted through holes in the mesh base. Synthetic fiber is the most popular type of hair prosthesis for women experiencing temporary hair loss because they are light weight, easy to adjust for fit, moderately priced, and comfortable.

Full-custom wigs have foundations that are made especially for the client by first making a mold and taking measurements of the head. The hair prosthesis is then hand constructed from this information to ensure an exact fit. Additionally, most full-custom hairpieces are made of human hair, making this hair replacement option as close to your own natural hair as you can get. They are also the most expensive.

3. How do you attach the wig to the scalp?

The feeling of security is the main goal when wearing a wig. Although a well-fitted wig doesn't usually require aids for attachment, some people like to have the feeling of additional security. The foundation, the material to which the hair is attached, should feel like a second scalp, and not be uncomfortably hot or heavy. In general, all wigs are warm, but some have special ventilation features.

The feeling of security is the main goal when attaching a wig to your scalp.

17

Using tapes and glues are the most common methods of attachment for mesh-based wigs. Practically every type of tape and adhesive known to man has been used, but the best and safest is a medically approved double-sided tape or toupé tape. The tape is applied along the sides of the mesh base. Once the wig is put on, it is patted into place, ensuring a tight seal between the tape and scalp. The tape is removed from the scalp with the use of alcohol or an adhesive remover (available at the pharmacy or wig supply).

Many women develop an allergy after repeated use of a tape. In these cases try using less tape and rotating the sites to which the tape is applied on a daily basis. You may also need to experiment with different brands of tapes. A commercially produced product called "Skin Prep," can help prevent or minimize the irritation from adhesives when applied to the scalp before affixing the hair piece. Additionally, French clips can be used if there are adequate amounts of hair in desired areas.

Some people are extra sensitive to tapes and other adhesives and develop burns. The best treatment for these burns is to keep the area clean and dry and allow the affected areas to rest (be tape/adhesive-free) for a few days. If the problem persists contact your physician.

When hair falls out the scalp may feel tender or sensitive. Since the base of many wigs can be irritating to the scalp it is often helpful to place a small cotton scarf or cotton skull cap between the scalp and the wig. Not only does the scarf or cap provide a protective barrier, but also absorbs some of the perspiration that develops on the scalp.

Suction is the newest way to attach a wig to a woman's

scalp. A custom-made plastic mold is made of the head, which is then used as the base for the wig. The hairs are often implanted into the form. The wig fits on the head without the use of adhesives. However, suction caps are better suited for people experiencing permanent hair loss rather than temporary hair loss, since as the hair begins to grow back in the suction effect is lost.

CHOOSING A WIG

Although nothing will ever make you feel as good as you do with your own hair, there is no reason why anyone has to know whether it is your hair or a prosthesis. The best way to avoid the possibility of someone suspecting a change in your hair is to get a wig as close as possible to your hair's natural color and style. Be sure to consider the length of hair you want to wear, since synthetic fibers longer than shoulder length may frizz from irritation against the body. For long hair, discuss with the wig consultant using human hair wigs or treating synthetic wigs with special conditioners to help prevent fiber damage.

If possible, before you lose your hair, cut and label pieces of hair from the top of your head, the side, and in the back at the nape of the neck. Take these hair samples, plus two pictures of yourself—one that shows the way you usually style your hair and another that clearly exhibits your hair line—to the wig salon or a hair prosthesis consultant. The specialist will take into consideration your skin tone, age, color of your eyes, the color of your hair samples, and the length and thickness of your natural hair. All these facts will help the stylist provide you with the best wig for you.

If you select a wig before your hair falls out, get a written guarantee that the price includes refitting the wig after you've lost your hair.

Test the fit by shaking your head back and forth several times. Bend over to see if the wig falls off. If possible, stand near a fan to see what the hair looks like after being in the wind. Can you see your scalp when the hair parts or moves out of place? Wear the wig for 20 to 30 minutes to see if it is comfortable. Like contacts it may take a week or two to get used to the feel of wearing a wig. In general, a wig should feel secure, but not binding.

STYLING WIGS

Styling a wig should be like styling your own hair—it should meet the needs of all occasions. Most wigs need fine tuning after purchase. It is essential to have your wig styled by a person who has had advanced training in caring for wigs. Find out if your personal hair stylist has had this type of experience (many do not) and if the stylist is comfortable with either synthetic or human hair (many may have a preference). Also, ask what percentage of their clients are women. The best source of information is referrals. Your local chapter of the American Cancer Society, cancer support group, or oncology nurse may be of assistance. In addition, they may know of funds available for women who need a hair prosthesis but cannot afford one.

Don't be afraid to be creative.

Often, taking the extra time and effort styling your wig will fool even more people into thinking that it is your own natural hair. Don't be afraid to be creative. If you have never used accessories in your hair before, this is

20

the time to do it. They are a very inexpensive way to coordinate your clothes and makeup, in addition to being fun to try on. By being inventive with clips, bows, scarfs, ribbons, flowers, combs, and jewelry, you will be making a personal fashion statement, perfect for all occasions.

CARING FOR YOUR WIG

The life of your wig will depend on how it is cared for, how much you wear it, and what it is made of. Just as with normal hair, chlorine, excessive exposure to sunlight, and blow drying will damage your hairpiece. Watch out for extremes in heat such as hot electric styling appliances, the oven, and the clothes dryer— they can melt or frizz synthetic hair. The following suggestions, in addition to the manufacturer's recommendations, will help preserve and extend the life of your synthetic wig:

Cleaning

Wash your wig about once a month or every 30 wearings in cool water with a wig shampoo (regular shampoo or detergents will dull the wig's color and may cause the wig to lose its shape and curl pattern). Gently swish the wig around in the water for about 2 to 3 minutes; rinse thoroughly in cool running water. Follow with special conditioners if recommended by wig manufacturer. After rinsing, drain off the excess water and then gently pat the wig dry with a soft towel. Do not use heat to dry a synthetic wig. Turn wig wrong side out and allow to dry completely, about 4 to 12 hours depending upon wig's length and density. Do not brush or comb wig when wet, or you'll alter the wig's original style.

Styling

When the wig is completely dry, brush or pick comb it back to original style.

Storage

Store wigs on a wig stand or a 2-liter plastic bottle. Don't use styrofoam heads as they tend to stretch the wig and tend to absorb odors which can permeate into the hair. Human hair wigs often require more care than synthetic wigs and are usually best cared for by a professional. All wigs should come with recommended care instructions which should include special shampooing and drying procedures, recommended hair care products, and styling guides. Always read these instructions carefully and review them with your wig specialist.

ABOUT INSURANCE

Loss of hair is considered by many insurance companies like the loss of a limb requiring a prosthesis, and as a necessary part of the rehabilitation process.

Loss of hair is considered by many insurance companies like the loss of a limb requiring a prosthesis and as a necessary part of the rehabilitation process. Insurance companies differ greatly from company to company and from state to state. Be sure to check with your insurance company to see if they pay for prosthetic devices. Your policy may list wigs specifically as an item for reimbursement, but many do not. Be sure to pay attention to exclusions. If you are unsure of what your coverages are, request a written explanation of benefits.

The first step towards getting reimbursed for a wig is to have your physician write a prescription for a "hair prosthesis." It is necessary for the word "prosthesis" to be on the prescription and on the sales receipt so the insurance company knows that this is not for cosmetic purposes. Many insurance companies still need to be educated about how the loss of a woman's hair interferes with her social and psychological well being.

It may be necessary for you to write an appeal letter to your insurance carrier to get reimbursement after denial of a claim. In your letter discuss the therapy you received and how it has affected you physically and emotionally. Outline the financial aspects of owning a wig on an annual basis—actual cost of the hairpiece, cost of styling, cost of maintenance products, and cost of repairs. Tell them that a hair prosthesis is just as necessary as a breast or a limb. If they pay for psychiatric help, explain that a quality hairpiece may eliminate the necessity of psychiatric counseling, thus saving the company money in the long run. If you are asking for coverage of an expensive hair prosthesis, explain why you have chosen that particular wig (other wigs make you itch, slip off your head, cause tape burns, etc.). Along with your letter and standard insurance form include the following items:

- Ask for a review by the medical board.

- Prescription from your doctor. Be sure he/she writes out a prescription for a hair prosthesis (not a wig) on an actual prescription form: "hair prosthesis due to the side effects of chemotherapy or radiation treatments to counteract psychological distress secondary to alopecia." The prescription should include your name and address. The doctor must date the prescription prior to your initial hair consultation appointment or hair prosthesis purchase. A brief letter of medical necessity from your physician or a psychiatrist may help.

- Ask for all replies in writing.

- Sales receipt. Have the salesperson write up a sales receipt for a hair prosthesis, and a description of it.

- A picture of yourself without hair. Many claims adjusters have absolutely no idea what women suffering from the side effects of chemotherapy and radiation look like. Many of the decision makers in the insurance business are men, who have little empathy with or real knowledge of the needs of women.

- A letter from your employer. Your employer should state that it is necessary for you to wear a hair prosthesis to remain employed, since coming to work bald is in violation of the company's dress code.

- Keep photocopies of your letter and all the paperwork you're sending.

Allow several weeks for the insurance company to reply. Insurance companies can be very intimidating and many are noted for giving their insureds the run around. Most states have "bad faith" laws, protecting insureds from their insurance companies. This law requires an insurance company to act within a reasonable amount of time in handling your claim. If you feel that you are not getting the service you are entitled to, write a letter to the insurance commissioner of your state, with a copy to your insurance company. The insurance commissioner regulates the insurance industry within each state. If your insurance company knows the insurance commissioner has been contacted, your claim will most likely be handled faster and more efficiently than before; however, it is no guarantee that your claim will be paid, so be sure to follow up. If the claim is still

denied you may want to consider taking your insurance
company to small claims court.

HEADWRAPS

The headwrap is perfect as a stylish alternative to a wig,
as well as a sensational way to accessorize any
ensemble. A headwrap can complement your looks,
enhance your style, and add versatility to your
wardrobe.

Making headwraps out of scarves is easy, but takes a
little practice. The emphasis should be on color and
texture rather than complicated tying techniques. For
beginners, it is helpful to purchase a mirror that you can
hook around your neck, in order to free both of your
hands. This type of mirror can be purchased at most
drug stores, variety stores, or beauty supply stores.

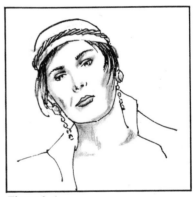

Figure 2-A

Department stores are filled with a variety of beautiful
scarves, but many are unsuitable for use as a headwrap,
especially for women experiencing total hair loss. The
following tips should make your selection easier.

- Choose cotton or cotton-blend scarves. Unlike silk or
  polyester, these materials will not slip off your head.

- For basic headwraps, choose 26-inch or 28-inch
  square scarves. You can use larger squares, up to 32
  inches for fancier wraps, and oblongs for headwrap
  trims.

- Fabric stores' remnants counters are a great source of
  inexpensive material. To make your own scarf, ask
  the sales clerk to cut the material into the desired
  size. Finish edges by turning in fabric to make a 1/4
  to 1/2-inch border on all edges; stitch.

Figure 2-B

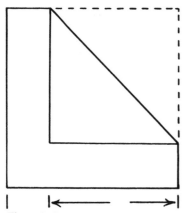

Figure 2-C

- Mix and match contrasting prints and colors by accessorizing with more than one scarf.

- Dress up a headwrap with ribbons, braids, twisted scarves, hats, berets, or jewelry. (Buy hats after you've lost your hair if you're not going to wear them over a wig.)

- Wash scarves according to the manufacturer's directions.

- Place a soft shoulder pad or scarf under fashion headwear to give a look of height and fullness.

Presented here are the step-by-step directions for a basic headwrap, plus several stylish variations. Once you have mastered these techniques, use your imagination and build on the basics.

BASIC HEADWRAP 1

Step 1 - Lay scarf flat; wrong side facing you. Fold scarf into a triangle, leaving one point slightly longer than the other (figures 2-B and 2-C).

Step 2 - Drape scarf over your head with the shorter side on top and points in the back. Pull scarf down until about two to three inches above your eyebrows (figure 2-D).

Step 3 - Tie scarf ends in a half-knot behind your head. The flap should be anchored beneath the knot (figure 2-E).

Step 4 - Tie scarf ends into a square knot (figure 2-F).

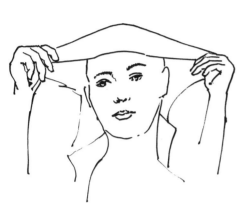

Figure 2-D

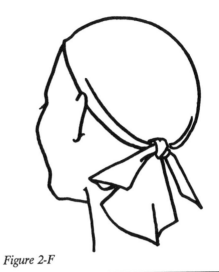

Figure 2-F

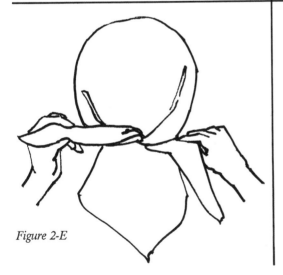

Figure 2-E

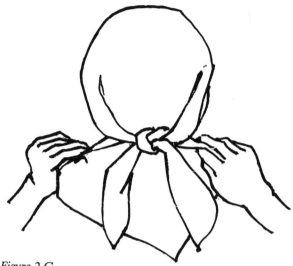

Figure 2-G

BASIC HEADWRAP 2

Step 1 - Perform steps 1 - 3 of Basic Headwrap 1.

Step 2 - Using both hands spread lower flap out under half-knot. Try to spread the scarf as close to the back of your ears as possible. If you are experiencing hair loss, this will help conceal that fact (figure 2-G).

Step 3 - Carefully bring flap up over knot and tuck flap and loose ends in behind knot securely (figures 2-H and 2-I).

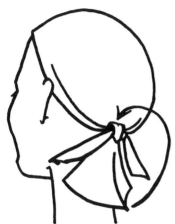
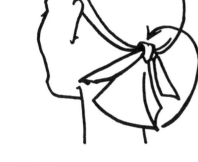

Figure 2-H

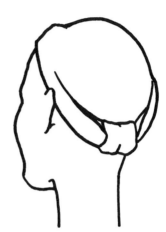

Figure 2-I

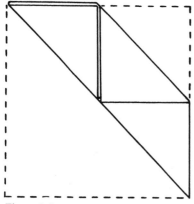

Figure 2-J

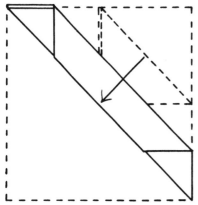

Figure 2-K

CONTRASTING TWIST HEADWRAP

Step 1 - Follow steps 1 - 3 outlined in Basic Headwrap 1.

Step 2 - Select a second scarf in a contrasting print or color. Lay fabric flat; wrong side towards you. Fold fabric into a triangle (figure 2-J). Fold top point down to bottom fold (figure 2-J).

Step 3 - Fold top fold to bottom fold (figure 2-K).

Step 4 - Take ends, one in each hand, and twist (figure 2-L). (For added interest, fold two scarves separately and twist together.)

Step 5 - Place twisted scarf over basic headwrap; tie in a half-knot at back of head (figure 2-M).

Step 6 - Bring ends of headwrap up over both knots; tuck all ends in securely (figure 2-N).

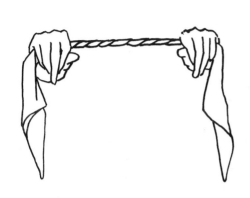

Figure 2-L

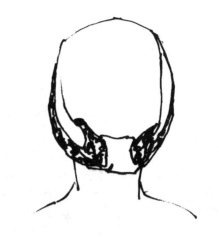

Figure 2-N

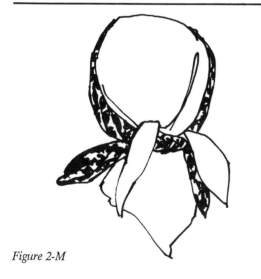

Figure 2-M

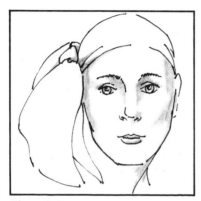

Figure 2-O

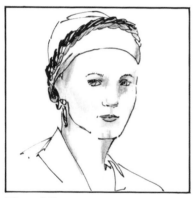

Figure 2-P

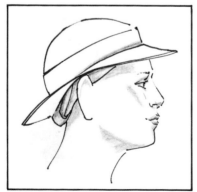

Figure 2-Q

BASIC SIDE TWIST

Step 1 - Tie Basic Headwrap 1 as described in steps 1 - 4, but place the knot over one ear instead of at back of head. Let the ends hang down loose (figure 2-O). For an interesting touch, add an earring to the opposite ear.

CONTRASTING SIDE TWIST

Step 1 - Tie scarf as described in Basic Side Twist.

Step 2 - Twist a second scarf as described in Contrasting Twist steps 1 - 4.

Step 3 - Knot; twist over headwrap above the same ear. Allow ends to hang loose (figure 2-P).

BASIC HEADWRAP WITH HAT

Step 1 - Tie Basic Headwrap 2 as described in steps 1 - 3.

Step 2 - Add hat of your choice (figure 2-Q).

SIDE TWIST WITH HAT

Step 1 - Tie Basic Side Twist headwrap according to directions.

Step 2 - Add hat of your choice, leaving scarf ends dangling at side (figure 2-R).

HEADWRAP WITH BERET

Step 1 - Tie Basic Headwrap as described in steps 1 - 4, but place square knot over one ear instead of at back of head.

Step 2 - Add beret, covering knot.

Step 3 - Tuck loose scarf ends up into beret (figure 2-S).

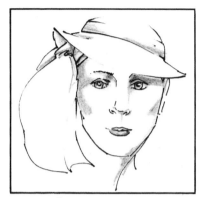

Figure 2-R

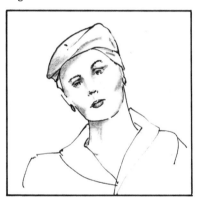

Figure 2-S

3
SKIN CARE

T he skin is the largest organ of the body covering about 18 square feet. It is composed of three layers: the epidermis - the outer layer, the dermis - the elastic second layer, and the subdermis - the fatty third layer. It is very sensitive, reacting to the internal changes (i.e., stress) in your body as well as to the environment around you (i.e., pollution, sun). In addition, it responds to diet, general health, age, stress, and heredity.

Cancer therapies can change the condition and texture of your skin, making it necessary to modify your normal skin care routine to accomodate such factors as increased sensitivity to the sun, increased dryness, increased oiliness, inflammation, loss of hair, increased facial hair, wrinkling, increased skin sensitivity to skin products, and increased skin pigmentation -- all possible side effects of chemotherapy and radiation. Additionally, some head and neck surgeries leave facial scars requiring special attention.

Cancer therapies can change the condition and texture of your skin, making it necessary to modify your normal skin care routine.

SKIN TYPES

Healthy skin needs regular care to stay in top condition. In general, there are four basic skin types -- normal, dry, oily, and combination. While no one has skin exactly like anyone else, knowing your skin type will help you design a skin care program to meet your individual needs.

Normal Skin

Normal skin is the ideal type and also the rarest. The woman fortunate enough to have normal skin has a smooth, blemish-free complexion that is neither oily or dry. Lines and wrinkles do not form until late in life. Good skin care will maintain its fine condition.

Dry Skin

Dry skin is characterized by its small pores and dull finish. Often dry and scaly patches appear, making it difficult to apply makeup. Expression lines and wrinkles easily form around the brow, eyes, and mouth. It is common for women to complain of their face feeling tight and chapped after washing.

Oily Skin

Oily skin is caused by the glands in the skin producing too much oil giving the skin a shiny appearance. This skin type is coarse textured with large pores and is prone to acne breakouts, blackheads, and whiteheads well past adolescence. You can not get rid of oily skin; you can merely learn how to control it.

Combination Skin

Combination skin is the most common type of skin for women between 25 and 40. It is characterized by moderate to oily skin on the forehead, nose, and chin (T-zone) combined with variable dry skin on the temples, cheeks, jawline, and neck. This type of skin can be cared for with a skin care program that controls oil in oily areas and adds moisture to drier areas.

TWO STEP SKIN CARE PROGRAM

When selecting skin care products, choose ones that you like and are inexpensive, fragrance-free, hypo-allergenic (little chance of allergic reaction), and alcohol-free for dry skin. Skin care products fall into two major categories -- cleansers and moisturizers.

Step 1 - Cleansing

The most important step in your skin care program is cleansing. Proper cleansing sloughs away dead skin cells and removes pollution's residue and makeup. These substances may clog skin pores, eventually leading to the formation of blemishes on even dry skin. Cleansing also stimulates circulation bringing an increased blood supply to the skin, leaving the skin looking fresh and alive.

The most important step in your skin care program is cleansing.

No matter what your skin type, your skin should be cleansed twice a day. Washing your face at night removes all the impurities that have collected during the day, including makeup and perspiration. A morning cleansing regimen rids the skin of oils that have collected during the night, along with any creams that you may have applied the evening before. Oily skin may benefit from cleansing several times a day.

There are many products available to cleanse the skin -- soap and water, creams, lotions, and granules -- each offering a different way to clean the skin.

Soap and water is the most basic cleanser. Oily skin types often prefer soap because of its drying effects.

Cleansing creams work by trapping dirt in a grease-like substance which then is removed with a tissue. Dry and normal skin types often select a cream based product because of its moisturizing effect.

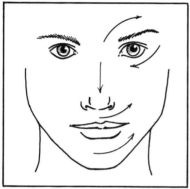

Figure 3-A

Cleansing lotions are a combination of a detergent and oil which is removed with water. Lotions work by loosening and removing surface soils, dead skin cells, and excess oil without stripping away the skin's natural moisture. All skin types can use this product.

Granules, also known as scrubs, lift embedded dirt and oil as well as dry flaky skin cells from the pores and bringing them to the surface to be rinsed away with water. Dry skin types can use a scrub once a week, while oily skin can use a scrub more often. Granules are not for everyone; they can cause irritation and redness. They should always be applied and removed gently. Granules can be used on dry patchy areas to exfoliate the dead cells remaining there. The body can benefit from the use of a scrub anywhere it is experiencing dry flaky skin. Simply apply the scrub to the affected areas and shower it off.

As a general rule, all cleansing products should be applied gently to avoid pulling the delicate surface of your skin. Further, if your platelet count is low, use extra caution to avoid bruising the skin. Always use an upward and outward motion (figure 3-A). With cleanser on your fingertips, start at the base of your throat, lightly stroking upward and outward. Continue by moving upward over your chin and jawline, around the outer sides of your mouth, nose, and on to the checks and temples. Finish, by working the cleanser upward and outward over your forehead to the hairline or scalp.

The area surrounding the eyes requires extra care. Always use your ring finger (it is weak) to lightly apply any product on this delicate skin. Below your eyes, move carefully inward from the outside of your eyes towards your nose.

To prevent damage, unnecessary wrinkling, and bruising, never pull, tug, or harshly manipulate any area of your skin.

Step 2 - Moisturizer

Moisture products are recommended for all types of skin to help your complexion maintain its optimum moisture balance. Moisturizers do not add oil to the skin, but act to keep you from losing moisture from the outer dead layer of the skin, plus some grease to hold in the natural oils. This step keeps the skin soft and supple, provides a protective barrier against environmental hazards such as wind and pollution, and helps makeup go on smoothly.

Moisturizers are available in two forms -- creams and lotions. Cost does not necessarily mean quality. The most effective body care products are "occlusive lotions" which remain on the skin's surface to seal in moisture. Some occlusives such as Vaseline can leave an unpleasant coat on the skin, so most people prefer lighter products. Choose the moisturizer that works best for you. In general, start with creams first, then move on to lotions. Be sure to read the labels; many moisturizing products contain alcohol which will aggravate dry skin. Oily skin may benefit from a light-textured, oil-controlling lotion that contains ingredients to absorb oil as well as to properly hydrate other areas.

Moisturizers are most effective when applied over damp skin.

Moisturizers are most effective when applied over damp skin. Gently smooth moisturizer over your throat and face every morning and evening after cleansing. Use light strokes following the same upward and outward movement of application for cleansing products.

SPECIAL CONSIDERATIONS

Blisters and Rashes

- Consult physician.

Dry skin

- Avoid alcohol based products.
- Avoid hot water.
- Use extra moisturizers.
- Exfoliate dry patchy areas with a scrub.

Inflammation

- Consult physician.

Increased Skin Pigmentation

- Use a sunscreen in addition to protective clothing.
- Discuss taking Vitamin B-6 supplements with physician.

Increased Susceptibility to Bleeding

- Be gentle when applying skin care products. Avoid harsh movements.

FACIALS

Facials relax the body and mind as well as cleanse the skin. They are the perfect way to indulge yourself once a week to reduce stress and make you feel beautiful. Facials are available at many salons, lasting up to 1 1/2 hours, but 20 minutes at home can achieve the same results. Regular use of a facial product helps remove dead skin cells and impurities, but more importantly, it allows a quiet time for you to relax and feel pampered. To prevent the skin from unnecessary trauma, choose a mask that washes off and does not require pulling off. Avoid products that burn or feel uncomfortable on the skin. If your platelet count is low, avoid scrubs which can cause damage to the skin and possibly subsequent bruising.

Dry and normal skins need a non-drying (alcohol-free), moisturizing formula, such as a hydrating gel or cream based mask.

Oily and combination skins will benefit from a clay based mask. Clay formulas absorb excess oil and exfoliate dead skin cells.

Masking products should be gently applied in an upward and outward direction over the face. Avoid the eye and mouth areas. Scrubs should be gently massaged into the face and left on until semi-dry, about ten minutes. To soften and relax the skin, place a clean, warm, damp facial cloth over your face; remove cloth when it is cool. Rinse your face with warm water, or remove any excess mask or scrub with a warm damp wash cloth.

REMOVING EYE MAKEUP

The removal of eye makeup requires as much care as applying it. In general, the two major considerations when washing the eye region are:

1. Prevent infections.

2. Prevent injury.

Since chemotherapy and radiation can make you more susceptible to infection and bleeding, it is important to use extra caution when cleansing the eye area. The best way to minimize eye infections and injury is to use disposable products (i.e., cotton balls) and avoid harshly manipulating the skin. Presented here are steps for the safe removal of eye makeup.

Step 1 - Dip a clean cotton ball into a non-eye irritating eye makeup remover of your choice. Apply eye makeup remover, by gently moving the cotton ball from the outside corner of your eye in towards your nose. Discard cotton ball after each motion. Avoid dipping the used cotton ball into the cleansing product.

Step 2 - Repeat procedure, one eye at a time, until makeup is completely removed.

Step 3 - Rinse eye area thoroughly with warm, clear water. Gently pat dry.

SCALP AND HAIR CARE

The health of your scalp and hair is as important to good looks as the condition of your complexion. Cleansing removes perspiration, soil, hair products, and other impurities that stick to your scalp and interfere with its functioning. Shampooing and conditioning your hair results in a fresh-smelling, lustrous, manageable, revitalized mane.

Although not all chemotherapy drugs cause hair loss, many can damage your hair, changing its type and condition. For example, oily hair may become dry and fly away. Chemotherapy can make your hair fragile, requiring extra gentle care when the hair is wet or dry. **Note that there are no shampoos, conditioners, or chemical treatments that will prevent hair loss.** Presented here are tips for caring for your hair while you are receiving chemotherapy to prevent or minimize hair damage or decrease hair loss when partial loss is expected:

Chemotherapy can make your hair fragile, requiring extra gentle care when the hair is wet or dry.

- Avoid excessive shampooing if you're experiencing dry hair.

- Use shampoos made for chemically treated hair (permanents, color).

- Minimize brushing and combing hair.

- Avoid use of electric styling appliances—curling irons, hot curlers, and blow dryers.

- Minimize use of hair sprays and styling mousses.

- Postpone receiving chemical treatments (permanents or color) until approximately 6 to 8 weeks after the completion of chemotherapy. Be sure to consult your physician first.

In order to cleanse your hair properly choose the appropriate shampoo for your hair type—thick, thin, coarse, and fine—and condition—dry to normal, or oily.

Shampoo

Dry to normal hair needs a gentle cleanser that removes dirt without stripping away oils and moisture.

Oily hair needs a cleanser that will remove excess oils along with soil.

To shampoo, wet your hair with warm water. Work shampoo into your hair with fingertips; lather shampoo and gently massage scalp with the balls of your fingers in a circular motion. Rinse hair and scalp thoroughly with clear, warm water, using your fingertips to separate strands of hair. Individuals with oily hair may need to repeat the shampooing procedure.

Condition

To keep hair shiny and flexible, all types of hair need a conditioner after shampooing. The scalp produces natural oils which seal moisture into the hair shaft. Moisture helps maintain strength. Conditioners supplement the moisture needed for dry hair and replace the moisture taken away by shampoos for oily hair.

After shampooing, gently squeeze out excess water from your hair. Work the conditioner into your hair, distributing it evenly up the shafts to the roots. Leave the conditioner on for one to three minutes; rinse hair with warm water until hair is smooth but not greasy. If you have extra oily hair, avoid getting conditioner on your scalp. Instead, work the conditioner up the hair strands towards the roots, stopping before reaching the scalp.

Gently dry hair by blotting it with a soft towel. Since wet hair is especially fragile and can be easily damaged, avoid harsh back and forth drying movements. Gently comb out hair.

Scalp Care

Similar to facials, scalp treatments combine massage with a mask and steam or heat. The goal is to cleanse the scalp, balance its natural oils, and deep-condition the hair. Just as every skin type benefits from an individualized skin care program, every scalp can benefit from the same type of treatment. When the scalp is healthy, the hair is healthy. Good scalp care has just as much value for the woman with no hair, since the problems of dryness, itching, and dandruff still occur.

Thoroughly cleansing the scalp and massaging it to stimulate blood flow may produce a healthier, stronger head of hair for women experiencing temporary hair loss. As the hair grows back in, maintaining this program can improve the appearance of dry hair by restoring its sheen. It is important to note that your scalp may feel extra tender following hair loss, requiring extra gentle care.

Scalp treatments attempt to get to the root of hair weakened by the sun, electric styling appliances, and chemicals. This type of therapy is available at many styling salons but also can be done at home. Dry hair requires monthly deep conditioning treatments which smooth damaged hair, followed by a stimulating massage to restore the oil balance of the scalp and result in natural shiny hair. Oily hair treatments require a mask that absorbs excess oils. Anti-flaking and anti-itching shampoos such as Neutrogena's T-Gel, can be applied for dandruff.

Scalp treatments attempt to get to the root of hair weakened by the sun, electric styling appliances, and chemicals.

Most treatments include steam phases to restore moisture. At home this is easily done by wrapping a warm to hot towel around your head while the conditioner is on your hair; remove the towel when it is cool. Heat treatments can also be used directly on the scalp if you are experiencing hair loss, but be sure to use a towel that is warm, not hot, to prevent burns since the protective covering of the hair is not there.

Our environment and lifestyle combine to damage our hair and scalp, just as they hurt the rest of our skin -- a little extra effort can make a big difference in how you look and feel about your appearance.

AGING

Women are fascinated with finding the fountain of youth. Many cosmetic companies claim to have the product that will reverse years of skin damage by wiping away wrinkles and lines. There are no creams, lotions, or other products you can purchase, or non-surgical facial treatments available, that will alter or decrease the wrinkling process.

Wrinkling should not be confused with dry skin. Dry skin can be helped with the use of a moisturizer. The change of the skin's integrity, elasticity, and structure is a natural process. Women are prone to wrinkles depending upon their skin type, the damage it has received from a lifetime of exposure to the sun and pollution, stress, and heredity. The best way to prevent premature aging is to minimize exposure to ultraviolet rays, use a sunscreen on all exposed areas of the skin when outdoors, keep your hands off your face, and maintain a good diet and exercise program.

A SAFER SHADE OF TAN

Beauty and health in our society are often measured by the darkness of a woman's tan. Despite warnings about the relationship of skin cancer to ultraviolet light, many people spend their summers baking at the beach and non-summer months in tanning salons or at distant resorts -- just to maintain their color.

While being in a sunny environment versus a grey and gloomy climate has been shown to be helpful in improving moods and attitudes, it is important to not be careless. While we are not suggesting that you stop enjoying the outdoors on sunny days, we do recommend that you follow a few guidelines. This is particularly important if you have had any radiation therapy -- the area treated is much more susceptible to sunburns and skin damage. In addition, certain drugs -- sulfa, tetracyclines, and some tranquilizers --, saccharin, and a few dyes can make your skin more susceptible to sun damage. Further, chemotherapy agents will also potentiate sunburning, and a sunburn can cause potentially permanent changes in the skin's pigment. These skin changes can occur during the time the drug is being given or can reactivate a previous skin reaction caused by sun exposure. Photosensitivity can be caused by the following chemotherapy drugs: actinomycin D, bleomycin, dacarbazine, doxorubicin (Adriamycin), fluorouracil (5 FU), methotrexate, and vinblastine (Velban).

Chemotherapy agents will also potentiate sunburning, and a sunburn can cause potentially permanent changes in the skin's pigment.

Often your skin will develop symptoms of burning, itching, and swelling when it is exposed to an amount of sun that normally wouldn't bother you at all. If you suddenly develop an irritation from sunlight, check with your physician to see if one of the drugs you're taking or treatments you have received could be causing the problem.

SUNBURN AND SKIN DAMAGE

People vary greatly in their susceptibility to sunburns and skin damage. There are two chief factors in determining how much damage a person will incur from sunlight:

1. The amount of protective pigment in a person's skin.

2. The amount and intensity of the sunlight.

Skin which produces large amounts of the skin pigment melanin suffer less damage. Fair skin burns easily, while olive skin has a greater tolerance to the sun.

Sunlight is most intense when the sun is directly overhead because fewer ultraviolet rays are screened out by the atmosphere. This is especially important during the summer months. Beware of the sun between 10:00 a.m. to 2:00 p.m. (11:00 a.m. to 3:00 p.m. daylight savings time). During these hours either avoid the sun or at least minimize your exposure and use a sunscreen.

The skin can be damaged even on hazy days because 50% of the suns rays that reach your skin are reflected off clouds, the ground or buildings -- not directly from the sun. Sand, water, and snow can reflect over 80% of the sun's burning rays. Consequently, skiers, sunbathers, and persons participating in water sports must use extra caution.

SUNSCREENS

Choosing a sunscreen has become a numbers game. Today, sun-blocking products have S.P.F. -- Sun Protection Factor -- numbers ranging from 1 to 29. Sunscreen products contain ingredients -- the most common is PABA -- that provide a barrier to the burning effects of the sun's rays. The amount of the sun-blocking ingredients determines the product's S.P.F. number. Each number determines the length of time you can stay in the sun before burning in the noon day sun. The higher the number, the greater the sunscreen's capacity to protect your skin from harmful ultraviolet radiation. For example, if before using a sunscreen it takes 10 minutes to burn, using an S.P.F. of 2 means it will take twice as long to burn -- 20 minutes. Using an S.P.F. of 20 means you could be in the sun 20 times longer -- 200 minutes -- than you could have without protection.

Using a sunscreen can be deceiving however, and should not be considered a license to increase sun exposure. The potential of skin damage is not eliminated by simply using a sun-blocking agent -- it must be used in combination with limiting sun exposure. Using a S.P.F. of 2 and staying in the sun 20 minutes, means the sun damage to your skin is the same as staying in the sun for 10 minutes without a sunscreen.

All types of skin, no matter how dark require some degree of protection from the sun. Choosing the appropriate S.P.F. number for you depends on your sun goals.

The potential of skin damage is not eliminated by simply using a sunblocking agent -- it must be used in combination with limiting sun exposure.

- If you want a tan and don't care about skin damage, use a low S.P.F. number (1 to 5).

- If you want a tan, but want to minimize the aging effects of the sun, use the highest S.P.F. available (currently 29).

- When in doubt, use factor 15 or greater.

INSTANT TANNERS

Several sunless-tan products have been recently introduced. They are designed for the woman who likes a tan but does not want to run the risk of sun exposure. Unlike bronzers which stain the skin, the ingredients contained in these products react with proteins in the outer layer of the skin (epidermis), darkening it within a few hours without sun exposure. The skin's color deepens with each application.

These instant-tanners are similiar to QT, which first appeared in the 60's. For most, the result is a natural looking tan, but for a few the skin turns an orangish color.

Pre-tan accelerators claim to speed up the tanning process by stimulating production of the skin pigment melanin. The manufacturers state that the active ingredient, tyrosine, allows a person to tan faster, so less exposure to ultraviolet rays is necessary. However, dermatologists dispute this claim by saying that the skin is impermeable to tyrosine, so accelerators can't work.

It is important to remember that most sunless tan products and accelerators don't contain sunscreen and do not offer any sun protection.

TANNING SALONS

Tanning salons have become the easy solution for the "me" generation to maintain a year round tan. Many individuals think they can keep a summer glow without risk by visiting the "electric beach".

Tanning booths are not safer than sun exposure. Ultraviolet rays are harmful to the skin, and it doesn't matter whether they come from the sun or an artificial source. In fact, tanning booths actually may cause more skin damage than natural sunlight, thereby increasing the aging process.

SKIN TIPS

- Know your sun type. When in doubt use S.P.F. 15 or greater.

- Wear sun block on all exposed areas of the skin.

- Beware of the sun between 10 a.m. to 2 p.m. (11 a.m. to 3 p.m. Daylight Savings Time). If you must sun at this time, upgrade your sunblock.

- Apply sunscreen at least every four hours, and again after going into the water.

- Wear protective clothing, such as a hat to minimize the hazards of the sun.

- Apply sunscreen to all exposed areas of your skin, including the tops of your ears, the top of your brow, the front and back of your neck, and your scalp.

- Know if any medications you're taking or have received will affect your skin's sun tolerance.

Ultraviolet rays are harmful to the skin and it doesn't matter whether they come from the sun or an artificial source.

- Locations at higher elevations and closer to the equator have more intense sun rays -- increase your S.P.F. number.

- Lip skin has very little protective pigment, so use lip block products.

4
MAKEUP

Makeup can produce miracles with the right colors and proper application. It can be used to accentuate your best features, be used as a camouflage, and detract from other features.

Makeup application is a skill that can be developed with practice, but often requires the experience and expertise of others. Treat yourself to a makeup consultation -- many department stores offer free advice at their cosmetic counters, but the best way to learn and get hands on experience is to see a professional makeup consultant. Find a consultant who will offer you personalized attention in a site that is private -- some consultants will come to your home. Question the consultant's experience with women who have side effects of cancer treatments. In some major cities there are makeup consultants associated with oncology clinics who specialize in the needs of women with cancer. Usually a session lasts approximately one to two hours and costs from $50.00 to $200.00.

The cosmetic industry is regulated by the Food and Drug Administration (F.D.A.). Unlike drug companies, makeup manufacturers can't make medical claims (i.e., their product will reverse wrinkling), but they can make a subjective claim (i.e., this product will make you beautiful). The code of federal regulations describes drugs as "articles intended for use in the diagnosis, cure, mitigation, treatment, or prevention of disease, and articles intended to affect the structure or any function of the body." Cosmetics are described as "articles intended to be applied to the human body for cleansing, beautifying, promoting attractiveness, or altering the appearance without affecting the body's structure or structure or functions."

Knowing the basics of makeup artistry is especially important for the woman who is experiencing some of the side effects of chemotherapy, radiation, and surgery. Changes in skin color can make you appear pale, washed out, grey, pasty, shallow, flushed, ruddy, yellow-orange, or tanned. Steroids can cause facial puffiness which often distorts features, and also increases production of facial hair. In addition to the hair loss from the scalp, radiation and chemotherapy can in some instances cause the complete or partial loss of eyebrows and eyelashes. Disfiguring facial scars are often the result of some head and neck surgeries.

Usually most of these situations can be handled with the proper use of makeup—changes in skin coloration can be hidden with under-foundation base toners, features can be redefined with the use of contour and highlighters, eyebrows and eyelashes can be filled in or completely reconstructed, and facial hair and scars can be camouflaged.

Makeup will change the way you feel about yourself and the way people will treat you.

Wearing makeup during your treatments is just as important as after you are through. Makeup will change the way you feel about yourself and the way people will treat you. Seeing a woman who has taken a small amount of effort—even if that means only lip gloss, makes those interacting with her feel more positive about her condition. These positive attitudes are infectious. If you feel good about yourself, others will too, and some of the fear associated with cancer may disappear.

The first step before putting makeup on is to thoroughly cleanse the skin (see Skin Care Chapter).

TOOLS

Although applicators are provided with most cosmetics, they are unsuitable for the look of a professional makeup artist. The quality can be poor, making them prone to falling apart before the product is used up. The tools needed for successful makeup artistry are:

1 - eyebrow brush

1 - lip brush

1 - makeup sponge

1 - fluff contour brush

1 - rouge brush

1 - translucent powder brush

2 - sponge tip eye shadow applicators

1 - dome eye shadow brush

1 - angle eye shadow brush

1 - eyelash curler

1 - tweezer

1 - pencil sharpener

cotton balls

disposable sponges

cotton-tipped applicators

All brushes should be made of natural fibers and sponges should be non-porous. Caring for these tools require washing in warm soapy water (Woolite is the best all-purpose soap), followed by rinsing in tepid water. Place tools on a towel and dry completely. To help prevent infections, make up tools should be washed at least once a week.

CHOOSING MAKEUP COLORS

Wearing the right colors on your face is as important as choosing the correct color of clothing. The right colors will accent your best features and add highlights and life to your face. Wearing the wrong colors can take away all facial definition, and accentuate features and skin pigments you're trying to cover up.

The color of makeup that will work for you depends on your skin tone and the color of your eyes. Skin tone is determined by the combination of three pigments -- melanin (brown), carotene (yellow), and hemoglobin (red). Two basic skin tones are derived from these combinations -- cool and warm. (For additional information regarding the seasonal approach to color, see chapter 5, page 89.) Your tone will determine the shades you'll pick for all your makeup. Although basic skin tones do not change with illness, they become more difficult to differentiate. Two women -- one with a cool skin tone and the other with a warm skin tone -- can have yellowing of the skin, but their baseline tone will make their discoloration look different. To avoid possible confusion and buying the wrong colors, try to determine your skin tone before you start treatment.

Although basic skin tones do not change with illness, they become more difficult to differentiate.

For some women, determining their skin tone is easy, but for others it is difficult. To determine your skin tone, place a piece of white paper near your wrist. Does the paper reflect blue (cool) or orange (warm)? If you're experiencing jaundice (yellowing of the skin) or redness you may need to compare your skin against others to get a true picture.

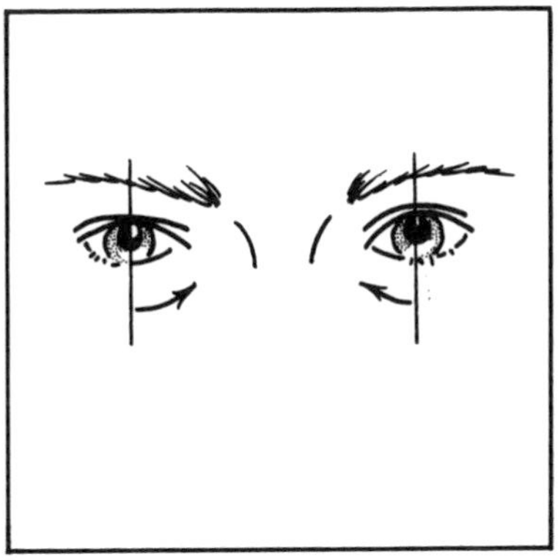

Figure 4-A

MAKEUP APPLICATION

CONCEALER

Concealers easily work to camouflage under-eye circles, blemishes, skin discolorations, and minor facial scars and abrasions. Formulated for your skin type -- cream for dry skin and liquid for oily skin -- concealers are available in three shades; light, medium, and dark. Choose a color that is about one shade lighter than your foundation or as close to your skin color if you are not going to wear a foundation.

To apply, dot concealer using a sponge tip or fine brush applicator over those areas you want to hide. Blend well using gentle upward and outward strokes. Take extra care with the delicate skin surrounding the eye, blending from the outside in.

The application of a light colored concealer in the eye hollow will offset natural shadows that fall there. Dot concealer starting at the center area under the pupil moving towards the inner corner; blend (figure 4-A). Follow with foundation, translucent powder, and blush.

If a general concealer does not provide adequate coverage try a peri-medical cream, such as

61

"Dermablend". Peri-medical creams are recommended by many plastic surgeons as a way to disguise scars. Apply as described above; blend well.

A properly applied concealer gives you the perfect base for your cosmetics.

HIGHLIGHT AND CONTOUR

Highlighting and concealing are based on the principles of using light and shadows to create some features and diminish others. Highlighters add light which can make selected features come forward and catch the viewer's eye. Contour makeup adds shadows to produce depth and angle.

Steroids are an important part of the treatment of some cancers. Their benefits can be great, but they are not without side effects. The most common include facial puffiness, fluid retention, increased facial hair, and increased susceptibility to infection. Fortunately, these side effects are usually temporary, and will go away as the steroids are tapered off.

When the face becomes puffy, its features can become distorted or hidden from view. Highlight and contour can be added almost anywhere to recreate and redefine facial structure.

Application can be tricky, so ask for assistance from a makeup professional while you are first learning this skill. Too much of either product can make you look like a clown, or even worse draw attention to an area you are trying to hide.

Highlighters

Highlighters should be two shades lighter than your foundation. Areas for highlighting include the brow bone, the outer half of the eye, top of the cheekbone, below the eye, and the center of the chin.

To apply, dot cream or brush powdered highlighter over the desired area; blend, working in an upward and outward direction until smooth.

Contour

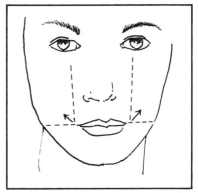

Figure 4-B

Contour colors are brown based. Choose one that is two shades darker than your foundation. Typical contour areas are the jaw, below the cheekbone, sides of the nose, temple area, and under the chin.

Facial Reconstruction

Cheek bones make the face appear slim and proportioned. To achieve the desired effect, set up boundaries on your face using your pupil, corner of the mouth, and ear as landmarks (figure 4-B). Contour should never be placed further in than the pupil or further down than the corner of the mouth. Your starting point is 1/4-inch up from this crossing point. An easy way to find your way is to suck in your cheeks until you pucker -- see the ridge? Along this ridge, using your landmarks as a guide, dot contour moving up towards the middle of the ear. The contour line should be no wider than 1/2-inch. Blend edges well so that no lines are visible. The starting point for under-cheek bone contouring is always the same, but the angle at which you brush up towards the ear depends on your desired effect. The steeper the angle of the contour

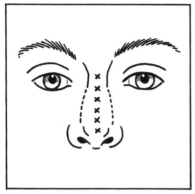

Figure 4-C

line, the longer the face will appear -- **perfect** for round steroid faces. A face that appears long and thin may benefit by aiming the contour line straight back towards the middle of the ear to give the illusion of a shorter, fuller face. Never place contour on the cheek bone itself.

Directly above the cheek bone brush highlighter, moving from below the eye towards the temple. There should be a space between the contour and the highlighter for the blush.

To create a thinner nose, first find your landmarks. Place your index finger flat down the center of your nose. Then lay a pencil along the side of it. Where the pencil lays is the area to be contoured. Run a line of contour down each side of the nose using a sponge tip applicator. Blend well. With another sponge tip applicator run a line of highlighter down the center of your nose. Blend well (figure 4-C).

A stronger jawline or chin can be developed by dotting contour along the upper edge of the jaw (for the jaw) or along the lower edge of the jaw (for the chin). Blend well, moving from the outside of the face in towards the chin.

Temple contour provides continuity with the rest of your cosmetics, so that your face color doesn't abrubtly end at your eyebrows. This is an especially important step for women without hair or bangs covering the forehead. As a result, applying contour in this area offers a way to achieve balance. Begin by dotting contour over the outer thirds of your forehead, starting from above the brow bone moving up to the hairline or scalp covering an area two to three inches wide on each side (figure 4- D). Blend well so that no lines are visible.

UNDER-FOUNDATION BASE TONERS

Under-foundation base toners, color correctors, fool the observer's eye into seeing your face with balanced, healthy skin color. Skin discoloration is a common side effect of chemotherapy and radiation. Color changes can make the skin look jaundiced (orange-yellow), sallow, ruddy, or pale/pallor. All these discolorations can appear to be reversed by applying the proper color of under-foundation base toner for each situation.

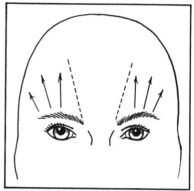

Figure 4-D

These color correctors are applied before your foundation, but after any concealers, contour, and highlight makeup you might need. Apply under-foundation base toner with a dry cosmetic sponge. Start by dotting each cheek bone, forehead, and chin with a small drop of toner. Smooth on evenly, using long, upward and outward strokes, working through the T-zone (forehead, nose and chin). Blend in at hairline and jawline to ensure a natural look (figure 4-E).

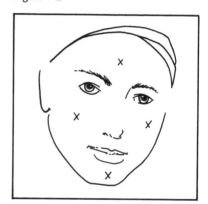

Figure 4-E

A variety of colors are available but this list should get you started:

> For yellow-orange skin use a purple under-foundation toner.

> For sallow, grey skin use a pink under-foundation toner.

> For ruddy, red-brown skin use a green under-foundation toner.

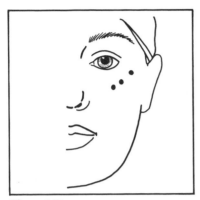

Figure 4-F

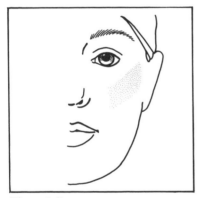

Figure 4-G

FOUNDATION

Foundation is a makeup base used to enhance the skin's color, even complexion flaws, and add balance and texture to the face. Foundations come in two basic undertones -- rose (cool) and yellow (warm). The best way to determine a product's tone is to compare one against the other. A rose base will have a purplish or pink cast, a yellow base will appear peach or yellow. Test a foundation's color by blending a drop on the jawline. The foundation should match your neck color -- no line should be noticeable.

Foundation should be applied over your moisturizer, concealer, and contour or highlighter (if you're using them). Apply foundation in the same fashion you would an under-foundation base toner (see page 65, figure 4-E).

BLUSH AND ROUGE

Blush can give a woman a look of warmth, health, and youth. When properly applied it can create cheekbones, add color, and diminish it. The most common mistake women make with cosmetics is putting too much blush on. Face color should be applied along the cheek bone, using the pupil, temple, and base of the nose as guidelines to form a triangle. Start by smiling, then move the brush from the mound of cheek below the pupil towards the temple, then move down along the ear until even with the base of the nose and move back to the beginning point (figures 4-F and 4-G).

Women with cool skin tones should wear a rouge in the rose family, ranging from blue-pink to burgandy, while those with warm skin tones need orange tones -- russet or tawny orange -- or delicate colors such as peach and coral. Be sure to coordinate blush colors with eyeshadows and lipstick.

Creamy rouge is best for dry skin, and dry powdered blush is best for oily skin. However, most women feel they have more control with a powdered blush.

FACE POWDER

Figure 4-H

Powders come in an assortment of shades, ranged by numbers, but the best for all-purpose use is a translucent, pressed powder. For very fair skin use a mid-ranged number. Lightly dust powder over your foundation and cream rouge, but before a powder blush, eyemakeup, and lip color. If you're experiencing extra-dry skin, you may choose to omit the powder. Also, to maintain a dewey look while you receiving chemotherapy, decrease your use of powder. As a finishing touch, powders are now available that help correct skin color -- for added luminescence and to conceal sallowness, use a purple (cool) or violet (warm) pressed powder; green powder diminishes the red in florid skin; and rose compensates for dull, pale skin.

EYE MAKEUP

Eyes are the focal point of a woman's face. Eyebrows and eyelashes softly frame the eyes. Eyeshadows highlight and accent the color of the eye. Portions of the eye are commonly used as landmarks for makeup application. To help you follow the directions for cosmetic application, figure 4-H names the various parts of the eye's anatomy. In addition to the eye's basic

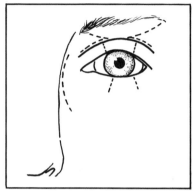

Figure 4-I

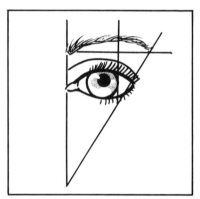

Figure 4-J

parts, it has been divided into makeup zones. Figure 4-I can be used as a reference for placement of color.

EYEBROWS

Eyebrow loss does not always accompany scalp hair loss due to chemotherapy and radiation treatments. When the brow hairs are affected, they may completely fall out or partially fall out leaving a patchy appearance. Presented here are the basics for eyebrow care, and techniques for reconstruction for fragmentary and total eyebrow loss.

The Basics

Eyebrows not only frame the eyes, but give the impression of the eye's length and width. The brow should begin directly over the inner corner of the eye. The thickest part of the brow should be in this area and should taper up to the middle arch. The arch's mid-point should be in line with the back one-third of the outer edge of the iris. The brow should taper down until in line with the outer edge of the eye. The beginning and end of the brow should be even. Neither end should drop lower than the other.

Using a pencil, it is easy to find the eyebrow's landmarks (figure 4-J). First place the pencil upright along the side of your nose. Your brow should meet the pencil, but not go past it. Next, hold the pencil at an angle so it intersects with the outer corner of your eye -- your eyebrow should end here. Now check if your eyebrow begins and ends at the same level by laying a pencil parallel to your eyes across the bridge of your nose. As the last step, hold your pencil upright so that

68

it is in line with the outer edge of the iris and the middle of your brow. The point where it intersects the eyebrow is where the highest portion of the brow should be.

An eyebrow is not a solid hard line of color over your eyes. It should appear feathery and full. An eyebrow pencil is used to add texture and shape. The color should either be as close to your natural hair color as possible or one shade lighter. Women with cool skin tones can select shades such as taupe, black-brown, or charcoal-grey, while women with warm skin tones should choose shades of brown. Black is rarely used for any skin tone. In general, the color of your brows should never be darker than your natural hair color.

An eyebrow is not a solid hard line of color over your eyes. It should appear feathery and full.

Before applying eyebrow color, brush brows with an eyebrow brush, using upward and outward strokes. Shade brows if necessary with light, short pencil strokes. Fill in any sparse areas as needed with the same feathery strokes. Again, brush eyebrows in an upward and outward fashion to blend natural hairs with pencil strokes.

To achieve a fuller look, use a slanted eyebrow brush and brush powdered eyeshadow (taupes and browns) upward and outward on the brow.

Tweezing

Tweezing is an excellent way to shape and thin brows. Eyebrows should be plucked so that the brow meets the guidelines you have set up. When you tweeze always follow the natural shape of the eye. Never pull hairs that grow above the brow. Remember, the eyebrow gives the eye a look of length and width. An eyebrow plucked too far away from the nose will **make** the eye look small. The eye will appear droopy if the brow's beginning and end aren't the same distance above the eye.

Before you tweeze, soften the eyebrow area with a warm, damp cloth. Hold it against your skin for about one minute; this opens up the hair follicles making it easier to pluck each hair out. Next, use a clean, dry pair of tweezers and pull out unwanted brow hairs one at a time. Do not tweeze the brows so that they become too thin.

If you are currently at high risk for infection or bleeding, it is best to omit tweezing. In these cases, use neutral tones of eye shadows so as not to call attention to your brows.

Eyebrow Reconstruction

Reconstructing eyebrows requires only following a few steps to achieve a natural look. It may take you a few attempts to feel comfortable with this technique, but with a little practice you'll be a professional.

The color of a person's hair is not all one color, but each strand is a shade of one basic color. Mixed together these values of the same color add luster, highlight, and personality to a head of hair and a set of eyebrows.

To recreate a natural appearing brow you'll need two eyebrow pencils -- one matching the dark value in your hair and the second matching the medium value in your hair. If possible, buy these pencils before you lose your hair so you're not relying on your memory. Saving portions of your hair (see page 20) or a good color photograph of you will help the cosmetic clerk help you select the correct shades.

The "dot-feather" technique can be used for filling in a brow with partial hair loss or to reconstruct a complete brow.

Step 1 - Follow guidelines described in eyebrow basics (page 68) for finding your eyebrow's boundaries. Using an eyebrow pencil place a dot to mark parameters (figure 4-K).

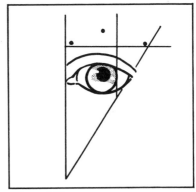

Figure 4-K

Step 2 - Alternately use the two colors of pencils you've selected, and mark the skin with light dots of color along the course you have developed for the brow (figure 4-L). The dots should look like a shadow, not a line.

Step 3 - Make one short, feathery stroke upward from each dot. Follow the brow curve. Fill in with strokes of color where needed (figure 4-M). The color should not be too light or dark, but conservative. Remember, the goal is to achieve a look similiar to your natural brow -- which includes being able to see flesh underneath.

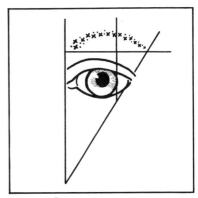

Figure 4-L

Step 4 - Lightly brush translucent powder over completed brow to achieve a set look, or use a brow fixitive such as "Brow Stay", which keeps the brow in place for one day.

Eyebrow Alternatives

Other options are available for women without eyebrows. The first is a prosthesis. Some wig manufacturers have developed custom eyebrows made

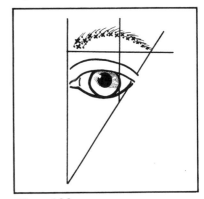

Figure 4-M

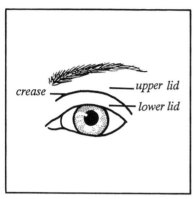

Figure 4-N

of natural European hair. They are simple to apply, only requiring a thin band of adhesive.

For women whose brow loss is permanent, micropigmentation might be the answer. Micropigmentation is a tatooing technique performed by a plastic surgeon or dermatologist for cosmetic purposes, in this case to give the illusion of a natural eyebrow. This procedure is not advised for women while receiving chemotherapy or radiation treatments. If you are considering this technique, be sure to consult your oncologist first.

EYESHADOW

The purpose of eyeshadow is to enhance the eye and the overall makeup scheme. Your selection of eye shadow shades will depend on your eye color and the size and shape of your eyes -- deep set, prominent, or normal. A light shadow can bring out an area, and a darker shadow can make an area recede.

The eye is divided into three shadow zones -- lid, crease, and underbrow (figure 4-N). The lid and underbrow are the major areas where eyeshadow is applied. The size of these zones will help you determine which color and tone go where. In general, the larger the lid the darker or deeper the color can be. The smaller the lid the brighter or more colorful the tones can be.

To bring out a sunken area or make a prominent area recede use neutrals rather than colors on the lid. A light neutral works well for deep-set eyes, while a darker neutral is best suited for prominent eyes.

Shadows are applied with sponge tip applicators or eye shadow brushes, using long even strokes. Start from the outer corner to the inner corner of the eye, overlapping each line of color to achieve a well blended appearance.

Lid

If you use a colored shadow, it should be placed on the lid close to the lash, using an eyeshadow brush. The shadow should be similar to your eye color, but in a softer shade. Your eye shadow should not compete with the color of your eyes. Sometimes a neutral shadow placed on a colored one will soften the effect. Older women should avoid frosted colors. Frosts settle in the creases, accenting the wrinkles they're trying to cover up. Women with darker skin tones should avoid iced colors or white based colors to prevent an ashy appearance.

Underbrow

A highlighter is a neutral color placed below the brow that gives the eyes an open appearance. Choose a color that picks up the glint in your eyes. Women with cool skin tones generally have a blue glint and should select silver based shadows. Warm skin tones require shadows with gold accents. White highlighter is never appropriate for any skin tone. Underbrow color should start at the end of the brow and move in towards the arch. Now, bring the color down to the crease.

Crease

The crease separates the two major shadow zones -- the lid and underbrow area. Contour shades can be added to the crease for a more dramatic appearance to the eye.

Contour colors are medium to dark. Apply with a eye shadow angle brush, starting at the crease's mid-point and moving out along the crease to the end of the lid. Move in along the lash line on the lid stopping above the pupil, making a "V". Fill in the lid with a color lighter that the contour shade. For a glamorous look, bring the contour shade down below the lower lash line, stopping below the pupil.

Eye Shadow Tips

- Blend shadows well.

- Select colors appropriate for your skin tone, seasonal color philosophy, and eye color.

- Older women should avoid frosted colors.

- Use neutrals to bring out a sunken area or make a prominent area recede.

- Women with darker skin tones should avoid metallic or iridescent colors.

- Black women should focus on warm jewel colors.

- Women with dark skin tones should avoid white based colors, it can make the skin appear ashy.

EYELASHES

Long beautiful lashes accentuate your eyes. Mascara is the easiest way to achieve this look. Mascara is considered by many women as the most essential part of eye makeup. It enhances your eyes by darkening and thickening the lashes to make them appear longer.

There are three types of mascara -- waterproof, water soluble, and lash lengthening. Waterproof and lash lengthening mascaras are often difficult to remove and as a result can cause eye irritation. Water soluble is the easiest to remove and the least abrasive of the various mascara types. Most types of mascara contain animal fat, which with age collect bacteria. As a general rule, discard your mascara one month after you have opened it to prevent eye infections, even if you are not at high risk for acquiring infections.

Discard your mascara one month after you have opened it to prevent eye infections.

If you are currently susceptible to infection due to a lowered white blood cell count (decreased number of cells that fight infections), are on steroids, are experiencing dry eyes due to the decreased or lack of production of tears, or have a history of eye infections, it is advisable to omit the use of mascara and use other methods to define the eye.

Apply mascara by looking straight ahead into the mirror. When removing the mascara wand from its case, in order to avoid breaking the brush and adding air that dries up the mascara, do not pump the brush up and down. Stroke your upper lashes evenly from the base to the tips, curling upward with the brush as you apply the mascara. Allow the mascara to dry and repeat with a second coat. Brush mascara to your lower lashes using downward strokes. Move brush back and forth across the lashes to separate them if necessary. Again allow the lashes to dry. Separate and unclump upper and lower lashes with the corner of the eyelash brush or an old, cleaned up mascara wand or tooth brush. Be sure to wash all mascara application tools thoroughly in soap and water at least once a week.

Never select a mascara color which is darker than your natural hair color. Here are some suggested mascara colors for each seasonal color philosophy:

Winter: Black (extremely dark eyes only)

Brown-black

Charcoal-grey (for grey hair)

Avoid red-browns

Summer: Brown-black

Brown

Charcoal-grey (for grey hair)

Soft brown

Avoid red-browns

Autumn: Brown-black

Brown

Soft brown

Spring: Brown-black

Brown

Soft brown

Red-brown

False Eyelashes

False eyelashes can add a glamorous touch; however, they are not the best eyelash alternative for most women. The most natural looking are individual clusters that are added to existing lashes. These individual lashes are a good way to supplement partial eyelash loss. They are easy to learn how to apply and with a good glue these lashes can stay on for weeks -- even in the shower. Fill in your natural lashes where needed, applying short lashes at the corner of each eye lid and medium length ones in the center positions.

Strip lashes can be used with natural lashes or when there are no lashes. Check the false lashes for an even curl and a serrated edge for a more natural appearance. You can serrate the edges by cutting the ends with manicure scissors. Check the adhesive band, the finer the better. In fact, some bands are invisible. For a dramatic effect that creates depth, use a colored band. This is good for an evening event.

Carefully apply a thin layer of eyelash glue to the adhesive strip. Place the strip as close to your own lashes, or where your own lashes would grow, as possible and press the strip into place. Use mascara to combine natural lashes with false lashes or apply it to the artificial lashes only. To minimize your risk for an eye infection, wash your false eyelashes according to manufacturer's directions after each use.

Reconstructing Eyelashes

When false eyelashes aren't an option, or you just prefer not to use them, the "dot-smudge" technique will recreate the effect of eyelashes. It can also be used with natural lashes and will eliminate the need for mascara.

Step 1 - Select an eyebrow pencil the color of your natural hair or lashes; sharpen before use.

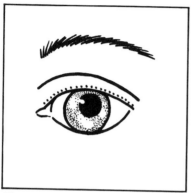

Figure 4-O

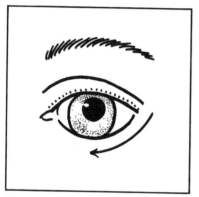

Figure 4-P

Step 2 - Dot the eyebrow pencil along the lash line (where the roots would be). Smudge dots with a sponge tip applicator or Q tip, moving from the eye's outside corner to its inside corner (figure 4-O).

Step 3 - Apply eye liner to lower lid, starting from the outside corner moving towards the center of the eye; stop just below the pupil. In general, eyeliners should be a neutral or smoky version of your natural eye color (figure 4-P).

LIP COLOR

Lipstick adds color to your face and pulls all your makeup together to achieve a balanced look. The colors you choose should follow the same rules you used for foundation and blush -- cool skin tones need rose colors and warm skin tones need orange colors. Your lipstick and blush colors should coordinate. The intensity of the color is determined by your skin tone, your personal preference, clothing, and occasion.

To apply lip color, begin by outlining your lip with a lip pencil. Lining the lips prevents the color from "bleeding" into the fine lines around your lips as well as defining the lips shape. Select a lip pencil color as close to the color of your lipstick as possible. Sharpen pencils to form a soft pointed tip for easier application. Line the lips following the natural contour of the mouth. Start at the center of the upper lip and use light strokes working toward each corner. Repeat on lower lip, first drawing a line in the center of the lower lip, then draw a line to each corner.

Lip pencils can be used to create changes in the lips'
appearance. Thin lips will appear fuller if you apply lip
pencil outside your natural lip line. Full lips will appear
thinner if you apply lip pencil just inside your natural
lip line (figure 4-Q).

Next, fill in your lips with color. Begin at the center of
your upper lip and brush color to each corner using
short strokes. Fill in your lower lip following the same
procedure, finishing with a clear gloss.

To decrease the number of lip color touch-ups, you
should fill in your lips with pencil before applying
lipstick. In addition, powders made especially for lip
color act to resist "bleeding". Lip powders are easily
applied using a sponge tip applicator.

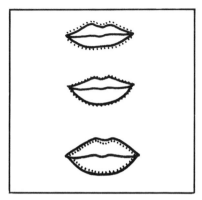

Figure 4-Q

SPECIAL CONSIDERATIONS

Jaundice

Jaundice is a condition caused by abnormal liver
function. The liver, considered the sewer system of the
body, processes most of the toxins and drugs that enter
the body. When the liver is damaged or its blood supply
is interrupted, it can not function properly and as a
result toxins such as bile, build up in the system. Often
alteration in liver function is noted by an orange-yellow
discoloration (icteric) to the skin, and the white portion
of the eye (sclera) becomes yellow. The skin may also
become itchy.

To draw attention away from discolored eyes and to
camouflage changes in the skin's color, choose colors
appropriate for your skin tone. If you're experiencing

jaundiced eyes, avoid green, purple, or blue shadows and liners. These colors will give a look of two black eyes. Instead, stick with neutral colors that bring out the color of the iris (the natural color portion of your eyes).

Skin with an orange/yellow appearance can be transformed with the use of a purple under-foundation base toner.

Facial Hair

The overproduction of facial hair is considered by many women as the worst side effect of steroids. Although some women naturally produce too much of certain hormones causing increase facial hair, it is important. that you discuss with your physician any thoughts about having your hair removed by any method -- waxing, electrolysis, or even having the hair bleached. Steroids can make you more susceptible to infections, and hair removal techniques may cause potential sources for infections to occur. Additionally, prior treatments, such as radiation, may have made your skin too sensitive for waxing or hair removal creams and lotions. If your oncologist gives the okay for facial hair removal, please have a dermatolgist do it.

The safest way to deal with facial hair is to camouflage it.

The safest way to deal with facial hair is to camouflage it. First, using your eyebrow brush, brush facial hair down so it is laying flat. Next cover hair with a concealer. Avoid applying powder over the concealer as the powder will accentuate the hair you are trying to cover up.

Scars

Whenever the skin is damaged, it is repaired by scar tissue. Scar tissue is formed by special cells called fibroblasts that manufacture collagen and other protein substances. The material produced is stronger and tougher than ordinary skin. Scars can vary in their appearance depending upon their location, your race, or age.

Before putting any makeup on a scar be sure that the sutures are removed, it is completely healed, there are no visible openings along or around the suture line, and there are no signs of redness, swelling, tenderness, or drainage. Also, check with your physician or surgeon to see if there any products you should avoid using.

A scar's type and location will determine its makeup needs. For facial scars, you may want to use some contour cream and highlighter at strategic places to draw attention away from the scarred area, or use a concealer or peri-medical cream (i.e., Dermablend) directly on the scar to camouflage it. Follow with foundation, powder, blush, and eye makeup. If the scar is on your lower cheek or jaw, you may want to spend extra time accenting your eyes. Conversely, if the scar is near your eyes or on your forehead, bring the focus down to the bottom half of your face.

A scar's type and location will determine its makeup needs.

In addition to facial scars, this information can be applied to body scars that you would like to conceal in order to give you more freedom in the selection of clothing. Apply foundation to scarred area; blend well so no lines show. Using a body brush, dust powder over affected area to set makeup so foundation will not get onto clothes.

Petechiae and Bruising

Chemotherapy may interfere with the body's ability to produce platelets. The reduction in the number of platelets (thrombocytopenia) circulating in your body may affect your blood's ability to clot resulting in bleeding. When this condition occurs, bleeding can start anywhere -- the mouth, gut, skin, and eyes -- but early signs of low platelets is commonly seen in the skin with the appearance of small scattered red dots (petechiae) or bruises (ecchymosis) on the arms and legs.

Petechiae, often referred to as pin point hemorrhages, form directly beneath the skin. In order to draw attention away from the affected areas, it is better to diffuse the redness rather than cover it up. A medium to thick foundation base will provide a believable skin-like finish (see page 66 for choosing foundation colors). Apply foundation with a dry cosmetic sponge. Start with a small drop of foundation over the affected area; blend edges evenly.

Bruises can be camouflaged with the use of a body bronzing or tanning gel. Begin by dotting preferred product over bruised area using a dry cosmetic sponge; blend edges evenly. In addition, bruises with a yellowish cast should be dusted with a tinted powder using a big body brush.

60 Second Makeover

It isn't necessary to go through all the steps of makeup application to achieve a healthy look. When you want a quick pick-me-up, dust your face with purple or violet powder and follow with lip gloss. In less than 60 seconds you'll feel better about your appearance.

SPECIAL MAKEUP TIPS

Jaundice

- Avoid green, purple, or blue eyeshadows and liners.

- Use neutral eyeshadow colors.

- Use purple under-foundation base toner.

Steroids

- For facial puffiness use contour creams and highlighters to create and redefine features.

- For facial hair, brush hair down and cover with concealer.

Ruddy Skin

- Use red-brown under-foundation base toner.

        or

- Dust on green pressed powder.

Sallow Skin

- Use pink under-foundation base toner.

        or

- Dust on purple or violet pressed powder.

Pale Skin

- Dust on rose pressed powder.

Facial Scars

- Use peri-medical creams on scars.

- Use contour cream around scarred area to lead away viewer's eye.

Body Scars

- Apply foundation over scarred areas; dust with powder.

Petechiae and Bruises

- Diffuse petechiae by applying a medium to thick foundation over affected areas.

- Apply bronzing or tanning gel over bruises.

PERSONAL MAKEUP GUIDE

Product	Color	Brand
Concealer		
Highlighter		
Contour		
Under-Foundation		
Base Toner		
Foundation		
Blush/Rouge		
Face Powder		
Eyebrow Pencil		
Eye Shadows		
Mascara		
Eyeliner		
Lip Pencil		
Lip Color		

5
CLOTHING

Women who feel good about their appearance also have a confident and positive self image.

C lothing can make powerful statements about a woman's personality, lifestyle, and attitudes. Although clothing needs may change after surgery due to the removal of tissue or the placement of tubes or bags (appliances) outside the body, it should not interfere with your ability to be fashionable and look your best. Women who feel good about their appearance also have a confident and positive self image. Wardrobe planning requires the analysis of four key components -- color, body proportion, personality, and lifestyle. Together these principles will give you the permission to be yourself and make a personal fashion statement. Every woman's taste in clothing is different. The styles of clothes you'll wear can be determined after you know your colors.

COLORS

Choosing your favorite color is easy, but selecting the right color to effectively improve your appearance can be difficult. Color can influence your moods, communicate to others the way they should feel about you, and provide the groundwork for an organized wardrobe. Wearing the right color can make you feel excited, powerful, motivated, and positive.

Color planning has been divided into four seasons -- Winter, Summer, Spring, and Autumn. Your skin tone, eye color, and natural hair color will place you into one of these four seasons.

While eye color and hair color offer clues in determining your season, the most important factor is skin tone. Skin tones are categorized as cool or warm.

Women with cool tones -- Winter and Summer -- have a blue undertone with a purple base, while warm tones -- Spring and Autumn -- have a yellow undertone with a green base. During periods of illness your basic skin tone does not change, but any skin discolorations can make it more difficult to choose the right colors. If possible, figure out what season you are in before you start your cancer treatments. (See chapter 4, page 60 for a discussion on how to determine your skin tone.) Wearing the wrong colors can make you look sick even when you're not, so selecting the correct one is even more important when you are experiencing the side effects of your therapy.

The seasonal color philosophy was inspired over 50 years ago by the European artist, Johannes Itten. He discovered that many of his students chose to paint with colors that complimented their individual skin tone, eye color, and hair color. In general, these colors fell into four categories, each unique in shade and intensity. He labeled each color palette after the seasons. The use of seasonal color plans have been expanded to be used as a tool to develop a wardrobe and makeup guide.

Winter

There are more winters than any other seasonal type. A winter woman can come from any corner of the world, making their skin color range from porcelain white to olive to dark black. Most winters have dark hair -- brown to blue black -- and deep colored eyes. These women all have blue skin undertones, requiring cool, clear colors to look their best. Winters can wear all values of primary colors, but they must be clear and blue-based basic colors. This is the only season that successfully wears pure white and black. There are no orange tones found in the winter palette.

Summer

Summer is winter's cousin, both sharing blue skin undertones. A summer lady has hair color ranging from mousey brown to ash blonde. Her eyes are often blue, green, aqua, or hazel. Women in this category should wear the cool, blue undertones found in soft pastels to dusky dark tones. Colors in this palette are clear to powdered (muted), and less intense than winter. Light to medium colors can be clear or muted, but medium to dark colors should be dusky.

Both Winter and Summer women wear silver jewelry.

Spring

Women in the Spring color group wear yellow undertones that are warm, clear, delicate, or bright. Characteristic of Spring is shades of blonde to golden brown hair and blue, green, or aqua eyes. Spring has more color options than any other season, but can only wear shades that are light to medium -- never dark clothes.

Autumn

Autumn's colors share Spring's yellow undertones, but are stronger and can be found in earthy muted shades with hints of orange, and colors of metals and wood such as gold and brown. Many of Autumn's and Spring's colors seem to overlap so be sure to select the correct color for your season. An Autumn woman usually has red hair or brown hair with gold and red highlights. Her eyes are often brown or green.

The colors in Spring and Autumn look best if accessorized with gold jewelry.

SPECIAL COLOR SITUATIONS

Side effects of chemotherapy, radiation, and prolonged illness may cause skin discolorations making you appear pale, sallow (grey), jaundice (orange-yellow), or ruddy (red). The proper use of color -- clothing and makeup -- should make people notice you, not your clothing or changes in your skin. Remember, your baseline skin tone will not change from cancer treatments.

The proper use of color should make people notice you, not your clothing or changes in your skin.

Always choose colors within your season in order to correct the color or at least decrease the intensity of the discoloration in your face. Wearing the wrong colors will only make the situation worse. For example, if a winter woman wore orange it would make her appear sallow or washed out.

The orange-yellow discoloration (jaundice) of the skin can be the most difficult to down play. In general, colors should be chosen to make you sparkle. Here are some clothing color suggestions for women who are experiencing jaundice:

Cool Skin Tones

Winter and Summer -- violets, blue-violets, and purple.

Warm Skin Tones

Spring and Autumn -- periwinkle blue, blue-greens, smokey greens.

CHOOSING ATTIRE

Clothing can create the illusion of a well proportioned, balanced body with the use of line and design.

Creating an individually tailored wardrobe requires the analysis of your facial structure, body's proportions, height, weight, and special needs (i.e., mastectomy), in addition to season. Few women have a perfect figure. Clothing can create the illusion of a well proportioned, balanced body with the use of line and design.

The first step in figure analysis is to take an honest look at yourself undressed in the mirror. Stand up straight and make an objective assessment of your assets and flaws. Good posture -- shoulders back and stomach and buttocks tucked in -- will give you an accurate idea of how garments look on you. Slouching will ruin the lines of even the best designed clothes.

Concentrating on your assets, note your face shape, neck length, shoulder width, shoulder slope, bust size and location, midriff size, waistline size and location, hip size, tummy shape, length of arms and legs, and buttocks size and shape. Write down what you see. Knowing your body's proportions, sizes, and shapes will help you choose clothes that take advantage of your good points, and detract from your figure flaws.

Think of your clothes and accessories as having vertical and horizontal lines. The placement of these patterns will determine what the eye will see. Coordinating fashion's line and design with your body type will enable you to select clothes that will make the most of your appearance. Use vertical lines to add length and slim. Horizontal lines create width and add weight. These basic principles can be used in any area of the body to compensate or accent features. The goal is to achieve a balanced figure.

SPECIAL CLOTHING NEEDS

The treatment of cancer can make selecting attire a challenge. Steroids can distort facial features, while surgeries can create a body imbalance due to the removal of tissues (i.e., breast removal). Additionally, the surgical placement of tubes and bags (appliances) outside the body requires care in adapting styles to meet these special needs. Following the basic principles of selecting clothing, incorporated with the guidelines presented here, you will always be fashionable.

Steroids

Steroids can cause the face to appear abnormally round and puffy. In general, for extremes in facial shape, avoid repeating this design in your neckline. Instead, choose a contrasting neckline to balance your face. For example, a person with a round face should avoid round necklines and wear a "V" shaped neckline. Conversely, if your face appears to have lost a lot of weight and is thin and drawn, try a round or oval neckline.

Ambulatory Infusion Pumps

Ambulatory pumps, often referred to as "chemo" pumps are small drug delivery systems that provide an innovative and effective approach to treating certain types of cancers. This technology is also being used as a creative approach to symptom management and can actually prevent or shorten length of hospitalizations in many situations. Computerized pumps such as Pharmacia Deltec's CADD-series can be used to deliver pain medication, antibiotics, nutritional products, and chemotherapy.

Weighing about one pound, these sophisticated devices can easily be concealed in a fanny pack or small pouch. Although most of these pumps come with their own carrying case, most individuals feel that the cases look too medical in appearance and draw unwanted attention. Since these pumps are usually worn 24 hours a day for several days or longer, you should consider the following guidelines when choosing a carrying case:

- Ask to see the actual device that you will be using and the size of the drug reservoir. If possible, ask for actual dimensions.

- Choose a fabric that is waterproof and sturdy.

- Decide whether you are going to wear the carrying case around your waist or over your shoulder. Remember, you may be wearing this 24 hours a day, and having something around your waist may be less burdensome than over your shoulder. You may want to choose a pouch that allows you the option.

- Consider pump pouches as a part of your wardrobe's accessories. Have fun by purchasing a selection of colors, fabrics, and styles.

- Consider what type of venous access device (I.V. in your arm, Port-a-Cath, or right atrial catheter) you will have and where the tubing from the pump will be connected.

- Be sure that pump pouch zipper does not cut into the tubing.

- Select a style that allows easy access to the pump in case of an emergency.

Above the Waist Surgeries

The two most common surgeries for women that occur above the waist are the removal of breast tissue (mastectomy) or the insertion of a special tube such as a right atrial catheter or Port-A-Cath, used for easy delivery of drugs and fluids.

The right atrial catheter, also known as a central venous catheter (CVC line) or Hickman line, is a hollow, soft plastic tube designed to stay in place, dangling on the outside of the chest, indefinitely with proper care. Insertion of this catheter is considered minor surgery. The doctor passes the right atrial catheter under the skin and into a large vein until it reaches the entrance of your heart (the right atrium) (figure 5-A).

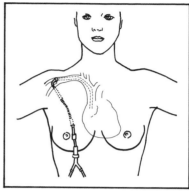

Figure 5-A

The Port-A-Cath was first introduced in 1983, and since then thousands of units have been implanted. The Port-A-Cath consists of two major parts—the portal and the catheter (figure 5-B). The insertion of the catheter portion of the Port-A-Cath is similar to the right atrial catheter, but instead of the end hanging outside of the chest, it is connected to the "portal" which is implanted under the skin in a surgically made pocket. In fact, having the Port-A-Cath completely hidden from view is considered by many women as its major benefit.

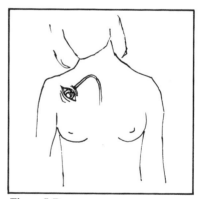

Figure 5-B

Neither of these devices interferes with the heart's function or normal activity. Instead, they allow easy access to the blood stream so that drawing laboratory tests and infusing intravenous medications (i,.e., chemotherapy), nutritional products, fluids, and blood components can be done without having to stick you each time with a needle.

The important dressing consideration for women with right atrial catheters or Port-A-Caths is to avoid any garment that might puncture or break the line (i.e., front clasping bras and pins).

The key to choosing attire if you want to hide, conceal,

95

or fool the eye into not knowing what's beneath above-the-waist garments is to follow these guidelines:

- Shoulder pads add balance to the figure by holding the garment away from the chest. This is ideal for the woman with narrow shoulders who has had a breast removed. Don't hesitate to wear shoulder pads with all your outfits, even your jogging clothes. Pads that attach to your shoulder can be purchased separately at most large department stores and many specialty stores.

- Soft fabrics drape best over chest appliances (right atrial catheters).

- To avoid puncturing the right atrial catheter wear a soft bra without an underwire.

- A bra's cut will be determined by where the right atrial catheter exits the chest or where the Port-A-Cath is located under the chest. Choose a bra that does not bind the catheter or cut into the Port-A-Cath.

- Scarves add a soft touch to a blouse and hide what is underneath. If your neck is short, avoid bulk, and wear a small amount of fabric close to the neckline.

- Try a cowl neck to hide catheters and add balance to a mastectomy. These necklines are becoming on all figure types. Be sure to note where the drape is placed—large busted women should be certain the drape is placed above the bustline, not on it.

- Select blouses and dresses with tucks, pleats, and gathers at the shoulder.

- Wide bat wing sleeves detract from chest area.

Below the Waist Surgeries

Disease, injuries, or birth defects that affect the normal functioning of the bowel (small intestine, large intestine, and rectum) or bladder may require a surgical procedure called an "ostomy". An ostomy allows body wastes to be evacuated via a surgical opening (stoma) made in the abdominal wall. The location of the stoma will be determined based upon which portion of the bowel is removed. A colostomy may be temporary or permanent. Some individuals with ostomies must wear special pouches (appliances) over their stoma to collect waste products.

There are several types of ostomy surgeries—ileostomy, colostomy, and urostomy—yet despite their differences their names are often incorrectly used interchangeably.

An ileostomy is often made as the result of the removal of the large intestine, often along with the rectum. The end of the small intestine (ileum) is brought through the abdominal wall to form a stoma, usually on the right lower quarter of the abdomen.

Colostomies are done at various points along the colon, so the stoma may be found on the right or left half of the abdomen.

Urostomies or urinary diversions, expel urine through an abdominal stoma instead of through its normal path from the bladder and urethra.

An ostomy should not limit your ability to look great.

An ostomy should not limit your ability to look great. Within the limits of your budget, try to expand your wardrobe. Many women with ostomies are better dressed than the average person. Following ostomy surgery, you may experience abdominal or perineal (vaginal area) tenderness for several weeks to months. During this time you may want to wear looser than usual clothes such as wrap around skirts and sweat pants. In addition, you may be using this period to psychologically adjust to your new body image. Most women with ostomies are self-conscious about what they wear, fearing that anyone who looks at them will know there is an appliance beneath their clothes. Thanks to the flexibility in today's fashions, and appliances that are slim and compact, women with ostomies can select clothes for all occasions. The secret is to wear clothes that avoid constricting the affected area and the appliance, plus camouflage what is beneath the clothes.

- Wear under-garments that come above or below the stoma, but not right on top of it.

- Avoid tight girdles or belts which rub the stoma.

- Suspenders may be more tolerable than belts, during the recuperative period following surgery.

- While getting used to a new elimination system, wear prints or plaids instead of solid colors so small accidents will go unnoticed.

- Buy trouser pants, the pleats in the front give extra fullness through the thigh and tummy. Choose soft fabrics with a drape such as silks, wools, and soft cottons. The result is a smooth, slim line with no hint of what is beneath.

- Full skirts made of soft fabrics work well to deemphasize the stomach area.

- Use accessories around the waist, such as belts and scarves tied on the opposite side of the surgical area, to move the viewer's eye towards the unaffected side.

- "Nude" stockings lack tummy control and are the perfect alternative to constricting panty hose.

MASTECTOMY

Practicality and fashion shape the post-mastectomy product market. Specialty stores are superior to department stores in alterations, privacy, and emotional support, as well as selection. In some cases the owners and/or sales staff have had mastectomies, but in all cases service is a priority. Atmosphere is a vital factor in creating a comfortable experience for the post-mastectomy patient. Look in the yellow pages under "Brassieres" or "Surgical Appliances", or contact your local chapter of the American Cancer Society's "Reach to Recovery" group for a list of stores selling breast prostheses. The average amount of time you can expect to spend finding a prosthesis and bra that fits is one hour. If at all possible, shop at a store that offers a variety of breast forms and post-mastectomy care products. Since every woman's body shape and surgery is different, no one brand can meet everyone's needs. In addition, you should be able to try on the breast prosthesis before purchase in order to ensure an exact fit. Buying a breast form by mail order usually ends up with unsatisfactory results.

Atmosphere is a vital factor in creating a comfortable experience for the post-mastectomy patient.

When breast cancer is diagnosed, two major treatment alternatives are available. One preserves the breast and the other removes the breast. Saving the breast (breast conservation) requires a lumpectomy (excision of the cancerous lump), removal of adjacent underarm (axillary) lymph nodes, and often several weeks of outpatient radiation therapy.

The surgical removal of the breast is called a mastectomy. There are three major types of surgery— simple, modified, and radical.

The simple mastectomy removes only the breast. Sometimes a few of the surrounding lymph nodes are also removed to see if the cancer has spread beyond the breast.

A modified radical mastectomy removes the entire breast along with the axillary (underarm) lymph nodes. Usually no underlying muscles (pectoralis major and minor) are removed yielding a superior cosmetic result compared to the radical mastectomy.

The radical mastectomy, the least common form of breast surgery done today, requires the removal of all the breast tissue and underlying breast muscles.

Lymphedema

Lymphedema is a possible complication following a mastectomy, caused by surgery or radiation treatments to the lymph nodes. As a result, the fluid from the lymph nodes circulates at a slower rate, impairing the body's ability to fight infections. The swelling associated with lymphedema can range from slight swelling of the underarm or shoulder to severe swelling and limited movement of the entire arm. Not all women develop this complication, but if swelling should occur, it is important to notify your physician immediately and take special steps to prevent infection. The degree of swelling you are experiencing will determine some of your clothing needs. In general, follow these simple rules.

- Avoid elastic or constricting cuffs on all garments.

- Wear watches and jewelry on the unaffected arm as much as possible.

- Avoid sunburns. Wear loose long sleeves or a sunscreen on exposed areas of skin.

- If shaving is necessary, use an electric razor with a narrow head for underarm shaving.

- Carry purses and heavy packages and bags on the unaffected arm.

- Wear protective gloves when gardening, cooking, and using harsh cleaning chemicals and detergents.

- Avoid garments or accessories that can constrict, bind, or puncture the affected arm.

- Avoid insect bites; wear insect repellant and protective clothing when necessary.

Unfortunately there is no cure for lympedema and it can become a lifetime problem. The good news is that it can be managed with the use of sequential pumps and custom-made venous pressure sleeves. The combination of these two devices used on a regular basis, as well as elevating the affected extremity when not active, is the key to successfully keeping this problem under control. Both the pump and the sleeves require a prescription from your physician. Many private insurance companies, in addition to Medicare, will reimburse a percentage of the costs for renting and/or purchasing this merchandise. A letter of medical necessity from your physician outlining the risks of untreated lymphedema (i.e., tissue infections in the affected arm) and the benefits of managing lymphedema will help you get insurance reimbursement.

Lymphedema pumps work by milking the lymph fluid out of the tissue and into the veins so that the excess fluid is brought back to the heart so it can then be distributed equally throughout the body. The most effective pumps are 12-chamber pumps, such as the Lymphapress. Lymphedema pumps are not recommended for everyone, especially individuals with congested heart failure, blood clots, or while experiencing an infection in the affected limb. Be sure to discuss using this device with your physician.

Venous pressure sleeves are worn to prevent and/or minimize the pooling of lymphatic fluid and subsequent swelling in the affected extremity. Ready-made sleeves or stockings will not adequately provide pressure where it is needed. Custom-made sleeves are constructed based on a series of measurements of the swollen limb. Your local post-mastectomy boutique or medical supply company can help you with these measurements.

The major terms used to describe women who have had

mastectomies which are necessary to know for fitting bras and prosthesis are:

Unilateral—removal of one breast.

Bilateral—removal of both breasts.

Reconstruction—replacing lost tissue due to surgery by the use of an implant or graft.

The loss of a breast is an emotionally and physically traumatic event. For many women recovery is not complete until they are made whole again. Reconstruction following a mastectomy is often delayed a few months, allowing tissues to soften and heal, but in some women it is being done immediately or within a few days of the mastectomy. In addition to the breast being replaced, nipples can be reconstructed by grafting pigmented skin from other areas of the body to the breast mound. To insure proper positioning of the new nipple, this procedure is often delayed a few months after the initial breast reconstruction.

BREAST FORMS

Following breast surgery, it is important for a woman to replace her natural breast weight in order to keep the body balanced. Unless the natural weight is replaced there will be an imbalance in the figure, causing one shoulder to drop downward and inward and the other shoulder to be up. In the case of bilateral mastectomies, the shoulders have a tendency to roll forward rather than stand straight, causing a rounded appearance. Back, shoulder, and neck discomfort are common problems when the body is not properly aligned. To prevent this lack of even weight distribution, all women who have had a mastectomy should wear a breast prosthesis. Additionally, a breast form will stop the bra from riding up or pulling to one side. There are a variety of breast

All women who have had a mastectomy should wear a breast form.

forms available, each designed to meet a specific need. Selecting the proper shape and size prosthesis will depend on two factors:

1. The type of surgery performed.

2. The style and size bra that has been properly fitted.

Breast implants don't have the same forward projection of a natural breast and don't fill in most bras. The result is that implants can appear lumpy or at a funny angle under clothing. Wearing a breast enhancing form, a partial silicone shell, can make a woman's implant look smooth and evenly placed, allowing both sides to appear natural. Also, many women find that bras made of a stretchable fabric look better over breast implants.

Today's breast forms are designed for active lifestyles and can be worn anywhere, even swimming. In general, a breast prosthesis can go anywhere you go. There is no right shape or placement of a breast form—whatever looks and feels best on you is the form you should choose. Breast forms can be classified in two basic ways: pocketed and self-adhering.

The traditional type of breast form fits into a pocketed bra or garment. This is the most common form of breast prosthesis available in the world. The newest type of form that has dramatically changed the post-mastectomy market is a form that adheres directly to the skin, requiring no special bras or a bra at all. The highest quality breast prostheses are made in the U.S.A., their workmanship is superior to others made in different parts of the world.

Leisure Forms

Leisure forms are non-weighted and designed for use on a temporary basis (sleeping, gardening, or leisure activity). A common cause of silicone breast form punctures are from rose thorns during gardening. Since the breast is not real, the woman can't feel the prick, resulting in damage of her expensive breast prosthesis. Made of polyester, cotton, or foam, leisure forms are not as heavy as silicone forms, making them comfortable enough to relax in. For women who have large breasts, lightly weighted leisure forms are available.

Usually it will take about four to six weeks after a mastectomy before a woman can wear a breast prosthesis for the first time. If you have ever worn contact lenses, you'll know that it takes time to get used to wearing them. The same is true for breast forms. You'll need to slowly build up wearing resistance to the form. Your chest wall needs to get used to having the weight there again. First, wear your form for one to two hours, increasing an additional hour or two daily until you're able to wear it comfortably for 24 hours.

Caring for Breast Forms

Caring for your breast form is easy. The prosthesis itself should be washed daily with a mild soap (i.e., Ivory bar soap or Neutrogena) and warm water. Rinse with tepid water and towel dry. Perspiration can actually permeate the back of the prosthesis causing the layers to separate, so daily care is essential. Many forms can be dried with a blow dryer, but be sure to read the manufacturer's care instructions for best results. Further, do not dry any breast prosthesis in the microwave. Forms without covers are often more comfortable if dusted with a body powder (avoid powders with talcum, oil, or fragrances) before wearing. Don't use detergents on any breast prosthesis and avoid lanolin-based soaps on the self-adhering style forms.

With proper care, the average life of a breast form is two years. A breast prosthesis usually will have a two-year limited warranty against workmanship and defects.

However, the guarantee does not cover punctures, so be careful of sharp objects (i.e., fingernails, jewelry, and pet claws) when handling and wearing your breast form. Further, always store your form in its original box or carrying case, or on a specially designed breast prosthesis stand.

BRAS

The key to fitting and wearing a breast form is a good-fitting bra. In general, a good rule to follow is whatever fits and supports the natural side, hugs the chest wall, and hugs underneath the arm and cup is the style that is recommended. Keep in mind that weight loss or weight gain will affect your bra size. A large variety of bras are available that provide comfort and security for the prosthesis wearer, as well as features to meet every need. Today's mastectomy bras are designed to look lighter and more feminine for the fashion conscious woman. Although surgical bras are more expensive than standard bras they do last a little longer. But, any bra can be made into a "surgical bra" by adding pockets. In many states "surgical bras" are exempt from sales tax, this is also true of breast forms. When your breast form begins to feel heavy when you are wearing it, this is an indication that your bra is losing its elasticity and needs to be replaced.

The key to fitting and wearing a breast form is a good-fitting bra.

All bras should be washed by hand in cold water with a mild soap, not detergent. Detergents will cause the elastics to deteriorate. In general, a bra will last about six months.

Bra Fitting

While many women will retain the same bra and cup size they had before surgery, it is important to know your correct size in order to insure a proper bra fit. Through the years a woman's natural shape fluctuates; making it necessary to check your bra size and fit at least once a year or every time you buy a new prosthesis. The major bra manufacturers all use specific sizing charts that correspond to your bra and cup size. The following steps will help you determine your bra and cup size:

Unilateral Mastectomy (one breast removed)

Step 1 - Measure for bra size. Using a tape measure, measure around the body directly under the breast (at the point where the natural breast tissue joins the chest wall). If the measurement (inches, not centimeters) is an odd number add 5 inches, and if it is an even number add 6 inches. The resulting figure is your bra size. For example, if you measure 30 inches around the body, add 6 inches. Your bra size will be 36 (figure 5-C).

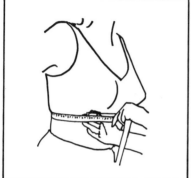

Figure 5-C

Step 2 - Measure for cup size. Have someone help you with this step. Put the bra on while bending at your waist to allow the breast tissue to fill the cup; then stand up and fasten. If this step is omitted the breast tissue will be displaced and you will not get an accurate measurement. Take a snug, not tight, measurement around the fullest part of your natural breast, from the center of the breast bone (sternum) to the center of the spine in back. Double this measurement (figure 5-D). For example, if your half body measurement is 18 inches, then doubled equals 36 inches. Compare this body size to your bra size. If this measurement is:

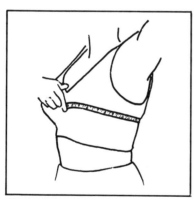

Figure 5-D

- The same as your bra size, your cup will be "A".

- One inch greater than your bra size, your cup will be "B".

- Two inches greater than your bra size, your cup will be "C".

- Three inches greater than your bra size, your cup will be "D".

- Four inches greater than your bra size, your cup will be "E".

- Five inches greater than your bra size, your cup will be "EE".

Step 3 - Measure fit of prosthesis. Put on a clinging knit t-shirt or silky shirt. The garments should have no pattern or pockets. Now look at yourself in the mirror and assess whether the high point (apex) of each breast are at the same level and that the slope and side contours of each breast are the same. Next, bend over to see if the form falls forward or stays in place as it should.

Bilateral Mastectomy (both breasts removed)

Step 1 - Measure for bra size as described for unilateral mastectomy.

Step 2 - A woman who has had a bilateral mastectomy can be any cup size she chooses. While many women stay the same cup size they wore before surgery, you may wish to wear either a smaller or larger size. The key here is to choose the cup size that will best compliment your height, weight, and figure.

Bra Fitting Check Points

- With your bra on, position form at any angle which most nearly matches your natural shape.

- The bottom of the bra, front and back should be straight or slightly lower in back. The straps should not cut into the shoulders.

- The bra should hug the chest wall smoothly, without gaping.

- No flesh should overflow at bra top or underarm area. All the breast tissue should be contained in the bra cup.

- The center seam should lay against the breastbone (sternum), without gaps between the cups.

- The cups should fit smoothly. Wrinkles in the cups on the surgical side may be corrected with darts. If the cup is not filled out, try on a smaller or light fiberfill style. If there is overflow at the top, you might need a larger cup for coverage.

- If there is pressure on the shoulders, you might want to try another size, the bra may be too small.

- The bra should close at either the snuggest or middle row of hooks.

- Back-fastening bras offer more breast support.

- Adjust bra straps for comfort and proper support.

- Check the nipple areas for even alignment.

- Check breast profile for even size.

- Most important, the bra should be comfortable.

For a perfect personalized fit, a bra must fit a woman's unique breast shape.

There's more to a perfect fit than just the bra size and cup size. For a perfect personalized fit, a bra must fit a woman's unique breast shape. Even if women wear the same size bra, they have different breast shapes. The silhouette of breasts and the amount of breast tissue varies from woman to woman. In order for you to select the bra with the best fit, look for one that meets your bra size, cup size, and breast shape.

Bra Care

Caring for your post-mastectomy bra is simple—just treat it like you would any fine hand washable garment. For best results, wash the bra in tepid water using a mild soap; air dry.

Mastectomy Accessories

Reconstructive surgery can leave the breasts uneven.
After-implant fitting aids are useful in achieving perfect
balance after reconstruction. Products are available that
will fill out any area of the breast to form a perfectly
contoured bustline.

Also, accessories designed for comfort and convenience
include shoulder cushions, bra extenders, sew-in form
pockets for swimming suits and bras, and artificial
nipples. Silicone nipples can be worn directly on the skin
or prosthesis.

Swimming Suits

Women who have had a breast removed can feel
confident and sexy in swimwear designed especially for
them. You'll look your best in a swimming suit with a
soft, scoop neckline or in a one shoulder type. Swimwear
with one shoulder covers the mastectomy side, leaving
the natural shoulder bare.

A swim prosthesis is recommended to be worn with
all bathing suits, although most brands of silicone
breast forms are safe in chlorine (be sure to check
manufacturer's recommendations). Swim forms are
relatively inexpensive, but will only last one season.
Depending upon your activity level, weighted—for
active wear—and non-weighted forms are available.
Chlorine will damage some brands of breast and swim
forms so be sure to check the manufacturer's suggestions
for care before use.

Wash swim prosthesis and bathing suit with a mild soap,
not detergent, and warm water after each use. Ivory bar
soap is best, since lanolin-based products eat away at
elastics and prosthesis materials.

Insurance

Post-mastectomy bras, breast forms, and accessories are often covered by most major medical policies. Regardless of when you had surgery, Medicare will pay a large percentage of the costs of purchase of a breast prosthesis and post-mastectomy bras. The amount of reimbursement and the number of breast forms and bras covered differ from region to region around the country. Contact your local Medicare office for a complete explanation of benefits. Additionally, if you have a back-up policy, this secondary or supplemental coverage will probably cover the balance.

In general, major medical policies pay for five-year replacements on the prosthesis only. Cancer write-on supplements to general health policies will usually pay for the replacement of a breast form. Many group health plans pay for the initial prosthesis and replacements as needed by physician recommendation. Health insurance policies differ greatly; be sure to read your policy carefully before making a claim. If you are unsure of exact coverages, request a written explanation of your insurance benefits.

HMO rules for prosthesis coverage vary from plan to plan. However, if you are on Medicare, the HMO must follow Medicare's guidelines when explaining your benefits to you. Don't feel limited by the referrals your HMO makes for you for post-mastectomy products. If you are unsatisfied with the referral, let your HMO know that you are not happy and wish to go somewhere else. Find out what they would pay the contracted agency or business and have that amount applied to your purchase at the establishment of your choice.

To apply for reimbursement, include with your claim form photocopies of the prescription for a breast prosthesis and post-mastectomy bra from your physician and the sales slip. Be sure the sales receipt indicates that you purchased a "breast prosthesis" and "post-mastectomy bra".

RADIATION RECALL

Radiation recall is a skin reaction which can occur when chemotherapy is given at the same time or following radiation treatments. The effects of this combination therapy can start several weeks after the radiation therapy has ended. Initially, the skin often appears red, similar to a mild sunburn, but can progress to include severe redness, swelling, tenderness or pain, blisters, and peeling—all similar to second or third degree burns. Additionally, after the skin has healed it may be permanently discolored on the areas previously affected. Several chemotherapy agents may cause a radiation recall reaction—actinomycin D, bleomycin, cyclophosphomide (Cytoxan), doxorubicin (Adriamycin), 5-fluorouracil (5-FU), hydroxyurea, vincristine, and vinblastine (Velban). If you think you are experiencing radiation recall, notify your physician immediately.

Caring for the affected skin area will vary depending upon the severity of the recall reaction. Your physician can provide you with guidelines for skin care that will meet your individual needs. In general your major considerations will be preventing additional injury to the skin caused by friction, pressure, or irritation, and keeping the area clean to prevent infections. The cosmetic effects of radiation recall can be devastating to many women, but the following tips should help you during the healing process.

Your major considerations will be preventing injury and infection.

- Avoid tight fitting clothes such as elastic cuffs, tight waist bands, bras, panty hose, and belts.

- Avoid irritating the skin with harsh fabrics such as

111

wool. Instead, wear lightweight fibers that can breathe (i.e., cotton).

- Wear loose fitting clothes such as big shirts, full skirts, and dresses with dropped waists.

- Minimize exposure of the recall reaction site to the sun (i.e., long, loose sleeves).

- Avoid swimming while experiencing a recall reaction.

- Avoid exposing the affected skin to extremes in temperatures, such as cold weather.

- Avoid shaving on the side of the recall reaction. If shaving is necessary use a narrow head electric razor.

- Avoid using creams and lotions not prescribed by your physician, or cosmetics, perfumes and colognes, powders, and deodorants on the skin in the recall site.

- Avoid wearing jewelry over the affected area.

6
NUTRITION
AND
EXERCISE

O verall beauty is more than the proper application of makeup and wearing the right colors -- a proper diet and daily exercise program takes care of the inside and shows on the outside. A well nourished, fit body can improve body image and feelings of well being. This chapter provides a nutrition primer and a work-out guide.

NUTRITION

According to the American Dietetic Association, more than one-third of all women in this country get fewer vitamins, minerals, and other nutrients each day than recommended. While good nutrition is important for everyone, it is especially important for the woman with cancer. Further, eating a balanced diet will make it easier to withstand the side effects of chemotherapy, radiation, and surgery by increasing the body's ability to fight disease, infection, and repair damaged cells.

Eating well means selecting a variety of foods from the four basic food groups -- meat, poultry, and fish; dairy products; fruit and vegetables; and cereal and grains -- since no single food supplies the approximately 50 nutrients needed for daily optimum health.

Nutrients -- protein, carbohydrates, fats, vitamins, minerals, and water -- are essential for building and maintaining body cells, regulating body processes, supplying energy, and helping the body defend itself against infection and disease. If one consumes the proper amount of the ten leader nutrients -- protein, carbohydrates, fat, vitamin A, thiamin, niacin, riboflavin, vitamin C, calcium and iron -- in the daily

Nutrients are essential for helping the body defend itself against infection and disease.

diet, the approximately other 40 nutrients will likely be consumed in amounts to meet body needs.

Protein, carbohydrates, and fats all provide the energy (measured in calories) to fuel the body. The body needs protein to build and repair the skin, hair, muscles, blood, and organs. Carbohydrates supply energy in order that protein can be used for growth and maintenance of body cells. Carbohydrates are the primary source of energy during vigorous exercise. In addition, they are essential for the normal functioning of many organs, including the brain, heart, and kidneys. Fat is the most concentrated form of energy, providing twice as many calories as protein and carbohydrates. When you are resting, fat is the primary source of fuel for muscles. Further, fat constitutes part of the structure of every cell along with contributing to maintenance of normal metabolism.

Vitamins and Minerals

Vitamins and minerals help the body use the major nutrients in foods -- protein, carbohydates, and fats -- so the functions of building and regulating can occur. Vitamins are present in the body in small amounts and are part of enzymes that regulate chemical reactions in the body. They are identified in two ways -- fat soluble and water soluble -- and in order to be classified as a vitamin, a deficiency must cause a specific disease. Simply, a fat soluble vitamin is stored in the body until needed, such as vitamins A, D, E, and K. All fat soluble vitamins consumed are stored, whether they are needed or not. A water soluble vitamin, such as vitamin C is used immediately, any extra is eliminated through the urine.

Some minerals are needed in relatively large amounts in the diet, such as calcium and potassium, while others are needed in very small amounts (trace minerals). In addition, some minerals may be required in greater amounts with your chemotherapy, such as magnesium with Cis Platinum. A balanced diet which meets the U.S. Recommended Daily Allowances (R.D.A.) for the vitamins: A (retinol), B (thiamin), B2 (riboflavin), C (ascorbic acid), and for the minerals: niacin, calcium, and iron will almost always provide the necessary amounts of other nutrients.

Using vitamin supplements may be required in certain situations. However, this should be based on inadequate daily intake, disturbed absorption, and increased requirements of body tissues. In many cases one multi-vitamin per day should be all the supplement you'll need to meet your daily nutritional needs (some interferences in absorption may require increased needs). Remember, taking too much of any one essential vitamin or mineral may show toxic effects and upset the balance and function of other minerals in the body. Before taking any vitamin supplement discuss it with your physician, since some can actually have detrimental side effects. Stress vitamins - the "super" vitamin praised by many health food stores is only necessary when there is a vitamin deficiency. The sales clerk can not diagnose a vitamin deficiency just by looking at you; it must be found from a laboratory test. To be safe, discuss with your physician any vitamin/mineral supplements you are considering to take. To make it easy to figure out what nutrients you need and their food sources, see table 1.

Some minerals may be required in greater amounts with chemotherapy.

TOP TEN NUTRIENTS (Table 1)

PROTEIN

Sources	Meat, Poultry, Fish, Eggs, Dried Beans and Peas, Cheese, Milk, and Eggs.
Functions	Forms an important part of enzymes, hormones, and body fluids. Repairs and builds all tissues. Helps build blood and antibodies. Supplies energy.

CARBOHYDRATES

Sources	Bread, Cereal, Potatoes, Corn, Dried Beans and Peas, Sugar, Syrup, and Jams.
Functions	Supplies energy so protein can be used for growth and maintenance of body cells. Carries other nutrients present in foods.

FAT

Sources	Shortening and Oils, Butter and Margarine, Cream, and Animal Fat.
Functions	Supplies large amounts of energy in small amounts of food. Helps keep the skin healthy. Carries fat soluble vitamins, A, D, E, and K.

VITAMIN A

Sources   Liver, Dark Green and Yellow
Vegetables, Cantalope, Butter, Cheese,
Whole Milk, Margarine, and Ice Cream.

Function   Keeps skin smooth and clear.
Helps keep mucous membranes firm and
resistant to infections. Helps prevent
night blindness. Promotes growth.

THIAMINE

Sources   Lean Pork, Nuts, Eggs, Dried
Beans and Peas, Whole Grain Breads and
Cereals.

Function   Helps promote normal appetite
and digestion. Contibutes to normal
functioning of the nervous system. Helps
the body use carbohydrates.

RIBOFLAVIN

Sources   Mild Cheese, Ice Cream, Meat
(especially organ meats), Fish, Poultry,
Eggs, Whole Grain Breads and
Cereals, and Green Leafy Vegetables.

Function   Helps the cells use oxygen in
order to release energy from food. Helps
keep the skin, mouth, tongue, and
digestive tract healthy. Helps prevent
scaly, greasy skin around nose and mouth.

VITAMIN C

Sources Citrus Fruits and Juices, Strawberries, Mango, Cantelope, Papaya, Tomatoes, Potatoes, Kale, Parsley, Greens, Broccoli, and Green Peppers.

Function Helps make cementing material that holds the cells together. Strengthens the walls of blood vessels. Helps in healing wounds. Helps teeth and bone formation.

CALCIUM

Sources Milk and Milk Products, Cheese, Sardines and Salmon with bones, Dried Beans and Peas, Citrus Fruits, Turnip and Mustard Greens, Collards, Kale, and Broccoli.

Function Helps build bones and teeth. Helps prevent softening of bones after menopause. Helps blood clot. Helps muscles and nerves to function. Regulates heart beat. Helps regulate the use of other body minerals.

IRON

Sources Liver, Red Meat, Fish, Egg Yolks, Dried Beans and Peas, Dried Fruits, and Whole Grain Breads and Cereals.

Function Combines with protein to make hemoglobin, the substance that carries oxygen to the cells. Helps cells use oxygen.

NIACIN

Sources Nuts, Dried Beans and Peas, Meat, Fish, Poultry, Milk, Mushrooms, and Whole Grain Breads and Cereals.

Function Helps keep nervous system healthy. Helps keep skin, tongue, and lips healthy. Helps cells use oxygen to produce energy.

WOMEN AND CALCIUM

Calcium deficiency is a major cause of osteoporosis.

Today, women are more aware of the existence of calcium than any other generation. Recent evidence suggests that calcium deficiency is a major cause of osteoporosis, a condition of weak bones. The gradual loss of the bone's structure begins in adulthood and progresses with increasing age. The problem increases after surgical or naturally occuring menopause.

Other factors that contribute to osteoporosis include:

- Lack of regular weight bearing exercise, for example walking at least three days a week.

- Hormonal shifts - after menopause there is a decrease in the hormone estrogen which causes calcium from the bones to be released into the blood. Prior to menopause, estrogen provides bone protecting/calcium conserving properties.

- Use of aluminum containing antacids.

- Smoking.

- Caffeine.

- Excessive protein intake (greater than the recommended daily allowance).

- Too much fiber from one food source. (It is best to vary your fiber sources from fruits, vegetables, and grains.)

Prevention

Prevention of osteoporosis begins during the teen years. Bones grow to their maximum strength only if a girl consumes enough calcium. The consequences of too little calcium during pregnancy and breast feeding may not be realized until later in life. Bones that have not had enough daily calcium replacements become fragile.

While a woman cannot undo years of calcium neglect, an effort at any time will help rebuild bones. Your recommended daily intake of calcium should be about 1000 to 1200 mg. It's recommended to get most of your calcium from foods if possible.

Calcium Supplements

Ideally, the calcium supplement you choose will have the highest concentration of calcium, be inexpensive, and free of chemical toxicants. Calcium carbonate supplements are the best since they contain the highest amount of calcium available to your body.

Antacids are a popular choice for calcium replacement, but they may contain aluminum, which stimulates calcium loss -- read the labels carefully. Avoid supplements from dolomite and bone meal which may be contaminated with lead. Also, if you have a history of kidney stones, check with your physician before taking any calcium supplements.

The Sunshine Vitamin

Vitamin D -- the "sunshine" vitamin -- is vital for the absorption of calcium in your body. When your body is exposed to the ultraviolet rays of the sun, it can process vitamin D. An adult can obtain adequate amounts of this vitamin through a balanced diet and exposure to sunlight.

Some calcium supplements contain vitamin D. Be sure not to exceed your recommended daily requirement of vitamin D (400 I.U.) between your diet and the supplement, since vitamin D is fat soluble, and too much can build up in your body and be harmful.

DETERMINING NUTRITIONAL NEEDS

No two women are identical in their nutritional needs. Your age, activity level, and state of health will determine your nutritional requirements. In general, your dietary requirements for all nutrients will increase 25% to 35% to meet your "stress" needs during cancer therapy and during the recovery period -- requiring extra calories and protein to repair tissues and recuperate. Conversely, a poor diet contributes to a poor reaction to stress and a slower rate of healing.

A poor diet contributes to a poor reaction to stress and a slower rate of healing.

To estimate the number of calories you should eat to maintain your body weight, first figure your ideal body weight. To do so, figure 5 feet eguals 100 pounds. Then add 5 pounds per inch, plus or minus 10%. For example, a woman who is 5 feet, 3 inches, should weigh 103 to 126 pounds, averaging 115 pounds. To maintain your recommended weight, multiply your ideal body weight by 10. Next, multiply your recommended weight by the activity level that best describes you: 3 for sedentary; 5 for moderate; and 10 for strenuous. Add these activity calories to your baseline calories. The result is the number of calories you need to maintain your recommended weight.

To figure your "stress" needs multiply your recommended weight by 30 to 35 for mild stress, 35 to

40 for moderate stress, and 40 to 50 for major stress instead of 10 as you did to figure your baseline calories. Add your activity calories to your stress calories. A registered dietician, pharmacist, physician, or registered nurse can help you figure your calorie requirements.

You may be looking at your baseline weight and thinking that your are either much heavier or lighter than recommended. Unfortunately, it is sometimes difficult to maintain good nutritional status because your disease and its treatments can cause symptoms that interfere with the desire or ability to eat a balanced diet. As a result weight may be lost or gained and the body's natural defenses weakened. A person is considered malnourished if their weight is 20% less than their ideal body weight (baseline weight). During periods where the body is literally starving its metabolic rate (ability to burn calories) is lowered in an attempt to conserve energy.

Your total body weight can be looked at as a combination of several basic parts -- fluids, bones and organs, muscle, and fat. The body's fluid balance is very sensitive and can easily change as a result of inadequate consumption of liquids causing dehydration. Chemotherapy and radiation often increase your body's demands for fluids making it necessary for you to be aware of the amounts you are drinking. The weight of bones and organs remains essentially unchanged during all states of wellness and illness, but the percentage of fat to muscle can change quickly with alterations in diet and activity level. Muscle burns calories -- determining how much you can eat. Anytime you become more sedentary, such as during periods of illness or stress, a percentage of your muscle turns to fat. In addition to the decrease in total muscle volume, the chemistry of the remaining muscle changes in such a way as to use fewer calories. Often you may not even notice a change in your actual weight, but only a change in your body composition. Perhaps you've experienced attempting to put on a pair of jeans that fit before your activity level changed and now finding they are too tight to zip up.

The body's ability to burn calories is like a car engine. When you put gas in your car, it's the size of the engine that determines the fuel consumption, not the size of the car. A small engine, needs less fuel to get around than a large engine. In general, the fat part doesn't need calories. In fact, fat loves fat. Fat is calories and doesn't burn them, instead prefers that the extra fat stay around. As a result, when a person begins eating again, weight gain may be quicker than expected with fewer calories consumed. When the body's ability to burn calories is reduced, it is like having a small engine that runs on less fuel.

Diet combined with exercise will reverse or slow down the process of muscle turning fat. In some cases you may need to eat fewer calories until your muscle composition changes so that it can burn more calories. When reducing calories do it without forfeiting the essential daily nutrients and considering your stress needs.

Diets

American women are obsessed with the notion that a perfect body is a thin, model-like body. As a result it is virtually impossible to read anything without finding another diet guaranteed to make you slim forever. It is very important, especially when deliberate weight loss is the goal, that you discuss the diet plan with your physician. Many diets do more harm than good, especially when undergoing cancer treatment. When choosing a weight loss program, always choose a diet that emphasizes a balanced selection from all four food groups. Participation in a group diet program gives many people a feeling of accomplishment from successfully completing a difficult task with the support of others.

Weight loss is big business, and every major city has many establishments specializing in diets. One highly recommended diet program is Weight Watchers. Their program is based on the American Dietetic Association exchange system, emphasising a safe balanced diet incorporating all the four food groups in combination with an exercise program.

Diets for weight loss or weight gain should be high in carbohydrates, low in fats, and low in protein. When intake of calories is too low the body must use the protein stored in the muscle for energy first, and there may not be enough left to repair body tissues. It may be necessary to increase proteins by 50% and calories by 20% during cancer treatments. Discuss any diet alterations and supplements with the dietician associated with your clinic or hospital and your physician.

Discuss any diet alterations and supplements with the dietician associated with your clinic or hospital and your physician.

Nausea, lack of appetite, and altered taste perception may make it difficult to eat. In many cases eating may have to be relearned. This is the time to establish good eating habits that will last a lifetime and not reinforce bad ones.

If you're experiencing taste changes due to alteration in taste buds, the following may be helpful:

- Try new combinations of foods.

- Experiment with textures, temperatures, and seasonings.

- Sugar tones down salty and acid foods.

- Salt tones down sugar and acid foods.

- Improve the taste of foods by marinating them in sweet juices, wine, Italian dressing, or soy sauce.

- Eating tart fruits with meals or using plastic utensils can reduce the bitter taste of foods.

Often eating the appropriate number of calories each day is easier said than done. Here are some tips to help you meet your caloric goals:

- Eat slowly.

- Eat frequent small meals, about four to six each day.

- Eat in a relaxed atmosphere.

- Eat in a pleasant atmosphere.

- Rely on food you really like.

- Experiment with different foods.

- Drink high caloric drinks as a snack.

- Try light exercise, such as walking before meals.

EXERCISE

Exercise is one of the simplest and most effective ways to utilize nutrients, build muscle, decrease body fat, reduce stress, and impart a feeling of well being. Dieting may decrease the weight of your body fat, but it can not increase the amount of muscle or reverse the badly altered chemistry of the muscles. Exercise increases muscle, tones, alters its chemistry, and increases its ability to burn calories. All three of the major forms of cancer therapy -- chemotherapy, radiation, and surgery -- require special exercise considerations. Chemotherapy's effects on your blood cells -- white blood cells, red blood cells, and platelets -- can change your exercise tolerance. Fatigue, commonly associated with radiation therapy, decreased white blood cells, and decreased red blood cells, requires low intensity exercise. Further, if you are experiencing a low platelet count it is important that you participate only in low impact exercises, such as walking, to prevent bleeding into your joints. In some cases, if your platelet count is less than 20,000, even walking a short distance can be potentially dangerous. Following surgery, depending upon the type of surgery and its location, it may be necessary for you to avoid certain types of exercises, such as heavy lifting, to prevent injuries. As you begin to recover from your operation, your surgeon can give you exercise guidelines and in many cases a complete exercise program. **Before starting any exercise program be sure to consult your physician.**

The safest and most natural way to health and fitness is just below your nose -- your feet. Exercise should become a part of your daily lifestyle. In general, begin

Exercise is one of the simplest and most effective ways to reduce stress, and impart a feeling of well being.

*Your body will tell you
what your limits are --
LISTEN, don't overdo.*

slowly with low intensity exercise, such as walking, before going on to more strenuous programs such as aerobic dance. When starting any exercise program, let your body be your guide. Your body will tell you what your limits are -- LISTEN, don't overdo. A good rule of thumb is, you should never be out of breath. You should be able to hold a conversation, but have slight difficulty forming the words. As your level of fitness improves you will be able to exercise more vigorously. When you do too much training, your body breaks down making it more susceptible to injuries and infections.

Aerobic Exercise

The most effective form of exercise is aerobic. Aerobic exercises are those that are steady and non-stop. They must push your heart rate (pulse) to 80% of its maximum for 20 to 30 minutes. Running, swimming, cycling, jumping rope, cross-country skiing, dancing, and rowing are all examples of aerobic exercises.

Your maximum heart rate (pulse) is the fastest your heart can pump and still pump blood to all your body's tissues. Nature determines your maximum heart rate, the older you are the slower the rate. To figure your maximum heart rate subtract your age from 220. To train your heart, and subsequent total body fitness, you must increase your pulse. Your training heart rate, the point your pulse should reach during exercise, is 80% of your maximum heart rate. For example, a 30 year old woman's maximum heart rate is 190 (220 minus 30 equals 190). Her training heart rate (80% of 190) is 152 beats per minute.

Some chemotherapy drugs can cause heart damage. In these cases, or if you have a history of heart disease, you should decrease your training heart rate to 75% of your maximum rate. In addition, if you are over 40 and/or have a history of heart disease and are just beginning to think of starting an exercise program, it is recommended that you consult your physician about having a stress electrocardiogram (EKG or ECG). The chart below (table 2) lists the recommended heart rates during exercise based on age and heart condition. Again, always consult your physician before starting any exercise program.

Consult your physician before starting any exercise program.

TARGET HEART RATE TABLE (Table 2)

Age	Maximum Heart Rate	80% of Max (Training Rate)	75% of Max. History of Heart Disease
20	200	160	150
22	198	158	148
24	196	157	147
26	194	155	145
28	192	153	143
30	190	151	141
32	188	149	139
34	186	147	137
36	184	145	135
38	182	143	133
40	180	141	131
42	178	139	129
44	176	137	127
46	175	135	125
48	173	133	123
50	171	131	121
52	169	129	119
54	167	127	117
56	165	125	115

Taking a Pulse

Taking a pulse during rest and exercise is easy if you follow a few basic steps. First, you will need a watch with a sweep second hand. You can find your pulse on the thumb side of your inner wrist. Take your pulse with the tips of your first two fingers, not your thumb (it has a pulse and you might get a double count). Move your fingers around until you find a strong beat. Sometimes it is easier to find a pulse in the neck. Gently lay your fingertips against *one* side of the neck -- one of your fingers will pick up the pulse. **Do not use your neck for finding a pulse if you have had any head and neck surgeries or conditions that might have disturbed the blood supply on either side of your neck.** Once you have found the pulse, count it for exactly 15 seconds. Multiply this number by 4 to get your resting pulse. During exercise, stop and take a quick pulse to get your training heart rate, then immediately resume exercising. Adjust your activity level up or down to meet your correct training pulse. Call your physician immediately if you experience symptoms of chest pain or dizziness during or following your work out. If your are feeling any discomfort while you are exercising, stop and rest.

Exercise should become a part of your daily lifestyle. The most important equipment you should buy is the proper shoe for your selected activity -- running, walking, or aerobic dance. It is important to start and end every exercise program with five to ten minutes of warm-up and cool-down exercises (i.e., stretching) to prevent injuries. The key to a good warm-up is to increase the pace of your workout so gradually that

Exercise should become part of your daily lifestyle.

133

your muscles can adjust to the increased pace and remain free of injuries. Likewise, cooling down allows the muscles to slowly relax after a vigorous work out and prevent subsequent cramping. Pre and post-workout exercises should stretch all the major muscle groups in the arms, legs, and trunk.

No two individuals are the same in their fitness needs. Physical therapists are available as consultants through most hospitals and clinics to develop an individualized exercise program for you. Further, you may want to join a structured group exercise program after your physician has stated that you can begin increasing your activity level. One of the safest exercise programs are the cardiac rehabilitation classes coordinated through your local American Heart Association. If you decide that you want to pamper yourself try a spa, but in either case, be sure to let the instructors know that you were recently treated for cancer so a program can be designed to meet your needs. It may be necessary for you to bring a note from your doctor indicating that it is safe for you to participate in an exercise class. **Following any surgical procedure, be sure to discuss with your surgeon and/or oncologist any physical limitations before restarting your exercise program or sport (such as swimming or golf).**

The rewards of maintaining an exercise program while receiving cancer treatments are a faster recovery, stronger heart and lungs, and continued emotional and physical strength.

7
MANICURES
AND
PEDICURES

Today's woman equates beautiful hands with long, freshly polished nails. If a nail breaks, she no longer has to wait weeks for it to grow back, but can go to the nail salon for a quick repair. Chemotherapy and radiation can cause damage to the fingernails and toenails which can interfere with their appearance and growth. Common changes in the nails include increased pigmentation making the nails appear darker, the appearance of lines and ridges, dryness, peeling, weakness, and slower growth. Chemotherapy agents often responsible for some of these changes include: topical BCNU, bleomycin, busulfan, cyclophosphomide (Cytoxan), doxorubicin (Adriamycin), and 5-fluorouracil (5-FU).

Chemotherapy and radiation can cause damage to the fingernails and toenails, which can interfere with their appearance and growth.

If you are experiencing dry, peeling nails, avoid alcohol based nail products such as nail polish and liquid nail polish remover. Further, acrylic nails can cause extensive damage to the natural nail and should not be applied during chemotherapy and radiation treatments. It is best to have artificial nails that use a glue as an adhesive removed prior to starting cancer treatments.

Well-groomed nails are even and smooth. In addition to caring for your hands and feet, manicures and pedicures are the perfect time for you to rest and relax. Everything you need for manicure is right at your fingertips. Maintaining well groomed hands only takes a few minutes each week by following a few basic steps. Keep in mind that your cancer therapy may have decreased your ability to fight infections (lowered white blood cell count) and increased your susceptibility to bruising and bleeding (decreased platelet count). In general, when doing a manicure or pedicure be gentle

All openings in the skin are potential sources of infections or sites for bleeding.

and careful not to puncture or nick the skin -- all openings in the skin are potential sources of infections or sites for bleeding. In addition, don't pull hangnails or cut cuticles. Most important, be sure to discuss with your physician guidelines for cutting nails.

MANICURES

TOOLS

Emery board

Cotton balls

Orange-wood manicure stick

Shallow bowl

Oil -- vegetable, olive, or baby

Hand lotion

MANICURE STEPS

Step 1 - Remove nail polish. Most nail polish removers are alcohol based and can cause damage to even healthy nails. Lanolin-based cream nail polish removers offer the best protection. Apply nail polish remover using a cotton ball; discard after each application. Be sure to rinse your nails thoroughly after using any type of polish remover.

Step 2 - Shape nails by filing them with an emery board. File nails in one direction only, moving from each side towards the center. Your nails should follow the contour of your fingertips, appearing oval rather than

square or pointed. Avoid filing in a back and forth
motion as this can cause ragged edges.

Step 3 - Soak nails, one hand at a time, in a bowl filled
with warm water for one to two minutes. Dry fingertips
with a soft towel.

Step 4 - Gently massage oil (vegetable, olive, or baby)
directly onto cuticles. Let oil sit on cuticles for about
one minute.

Step 5 - Wrap a cotton ball around the tip of an
orange-wood cuticle stick. Gently push cuticles back
with the cotton padded stick. Be careful not to tear or
cut the skin. (If you are at high risk for infections omit
this step.)

Step 6 - Rinse off oil. Dry hands completely.

Step 7 - Apply hand lotion to keep hands feeling soft
and smooth.

Step 8 (optional) - Apply nail polish. First apply a clear
base coat, then follow with two coats of nail polish.
Finish with a clear top coat. Allow nails to dry
thoroughly.

ARTIFICIAL NAILS

Acrylic nails are the most common form of artificial
nail. Although the cosmetic result is beautiful, the
damage to the nail itself is not. The adhesive used for
these nails cause dryness and peeling of the nail bed. In
addition, the chemical used to remove the acrylic nails
also promotes increased dryness and damage. This is of
particular importance if you are already experiencing

nail changes due to radiation or chemotherapy. In general, if you want to wear fake nails, select a product that uses a water-soluble glue versus a chemical adhesive. Also, be aware that excessive moisture trapped under artificial nails is a common cause of local fungal infections. In general while you are receiving cancer treatments and/or at risk for infection, it is best to avoid wearing fake nails.

PEDICURES

Your feet will most likely react to chemotherapy and radiation treatments in much the same way as your hands. Your feet, however, often require more care and attention. Since your ability to fight infections may be compromised and the circulation of blood to your feet may be decreased due to the side effects of chemotherapy, radiation, surgery, and other drugs and disease processes (i.e., diabetes), it is important to take care not to cut or puncture the skin covering your feet. Any break in the skin is a potential source of infection or bleeding. While you are receiving any form of cancer therapy, be sure to discuss with your physician guidelines for caring for your feet. In some cases it may be necessary to have a pedicure performed by a physician. The following steps are for an easy pedicure.

TOOLS

Manicure scissors

Toenail clippers

Large Basin

Oil -- Vegetable, Olive, or Baby

Body or hand lotion

PEDICURE STEPS

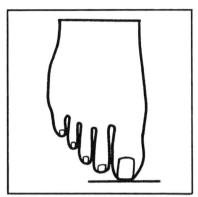

Figure 7-A

Step 1 - Soak feet in a large basin filled with warm water for at least ten minutes. Dry feet thoroughly with a soft towel -- between the toes too.

Step 2 - Gently rub oil onto cuticles. Let oil sit on cuticles for about one minute.

Step 3 - Gently push cuticles down with a soft towel. Do not cut cuticles.

Step 4 - Wipe all excess oil off cuticles and toenail.

Step 5 - Cut toenails square with a pair of blunt-edged manicure scissors or toenail clippers (figure 7-A). Avoid cutting nails too short (figure 7-B). Your toenails should be even with the ends of your toes. (Omit this step if you are at high risk for infection or bleeding, if the blood supply to your feet is interrupted, or if you are experiencing lymphedema in the leg.)

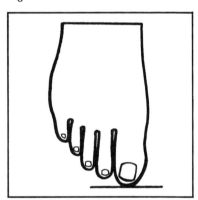

Figure 7-B

Step 6 - Massage lotion onto feet. Begin by rubbing lotion onto your toes, then work up over your soles towards your leg.

8
RESOURCES

Oncology nurses, social workers, and support groups and organizations are the best source of information for community and national referrals for services and products. The chapters in this book introduced you to a variety of products that provide solutions to the cosmetic side effects of cancer therapy. In general, makeup, skin care, corrective cosmetics, and nail care products are available in most major department stores or full-service beauty supply stores; wigs should be purchased from a specialist whose customers have hair loss related to cancer treatments; fashionable turbans and scarves can be purchased from hair loss specialists, accessory counters at major department stores (selection may be seasonal), and mail order; and following breast surgery, buy products from a specialty store that specializes in post-mastectomy care.

Just as you would check out the credentials of anyone providing a direct service to you, it is very important that you verify the credentials of anyone offering services related to your health, even if the person is a volunteer. Don't assume that because the person offering help to you is connected with a prestigous organization that they are qualified to meet your special needs. To save you time when interviewing an appearance/image consultant, use the following questionnaire:

GUIDELINES FOR CHOOSING AN APPEARANCE / IMAGE CONSULTANT

1. What are your qualifications and educational background?

2. Where is your business located?

3. Do you provide private consultation areas?

4. What are your business hours?

5. Will you go to a person's home or make hospital visits?

6. How long have you been in the business of servicing the needs of the cancer patients?

7. What training have you had that relates to the specific needs of the person with cancer?

8. What services do you offer?

   Does the person have a professional-looking brochure?

9. Do you charge an initial consultation fee?

   If yes, how much?

   Is it applied to purchase?

10. Do you help with insurance reimbursement for the items purchased?

11. What is your refund/exchange policy?

12. List at least three references.

Resources

Listed in this chapter are some ideas for products and services to get you started. We encourage you to support businesses in your community first, but depending where you live working with an establishment out of town may provide you with better service. If you were referred to a business, be sure to let the referral source know about the good and bad experiences you have had with the consultant.

SUGGESTED READING

BOOKS

Bailey, *Fit or Fat*, Houghton Mifflin Company, Boston, 1977.

Begoun, *Blue Eyeshadow Should Be Illegal*, Beginning Press, Seattle, Washington, 1985.

Benjamin, *From Victim to Victor*, Dell Publishing, New York, 1987.

Berger and Bostwick, *A Woman's Decision*, Mosby, Co., New York, 1984.

Bruning, *Coping with Chemotherapy*, Ballantine Books, New York, 1985.

Changes, Choices, and Challenges, Appearance Concepts Foundation of Canada, Toronto, 1989.

Cousins, *Anatomy of an Illness*, Bantam Books, New York, 1979.

Dollinger, *Everybody's Guide to Cancer Therapy*, Andrews and McMeel, Kansas City, 1991.

Duffy, *Hoax Fashion Formula*, The Body Press, Tucson, AZ, 1987.

Graham, *In the Company of Others*, Harcourt Brace Jovanovich, New York, 1982.

Gross and Ito, *Women Talk About Breast Cancer*, Clarkson Potter, New York, 1990.

Jackson, *Color Me Beautiful*, Ballantine Books, New York, 1980.

Jackson, *Color Me Beautiful Makeup*, Ballantine Books, New York, 1987.

Kalter, *Looking Up*, McGraw-Hill Book Company, New York, 1987.

Kashiwa and Rippe, *Fitness Walking for Women*, Putnam Publishing, New York, 1987.

Kauffman, *Surviving Cancer*, Acropolis, Washington D.C., 1989.

Kaye, *Spinning Straw into Gold*, Fireside, New York, 1991.

Kubler-Ross, *On Death and Dying*, Macmillan, New York, 1978.

Kushner, *When Bad Things Happen to Good People*, Avon Books, New York, 1981.

Margie and Bloch, *Nutrition and the Cancer Patient*, Chilton Book Co., Pennsylvania, 1983.

Maron, *Instant Makeover Magic*, Warner Books, New York, 1983.

Maron, *Makeover Miracles*, Crown Publishing, New York, 1993.

Mary Kay Cosmetics, *The Mary Kay Guide to Beauty*, Addison-Wesley Publishing Co., Reading, Massachusetts, 1986.

McJimsey, *Art and Fashion in Clothing Selection*, Iowa State University Press, Iowa, 1973.

Mirkin and Hoffman, *The Sports Medicine Book*, Little, Brown and Company, Boston, 1978.

Morra and Potts, *Choices: Realistic Alternatives in Cancer Treatments*, Avon Books, New York, 1980.

Mullen and McGinn, *The Ostomy Book— Living Comfortably with Colostomies, Ileostomies, and Urostomies*, Bull Publishing Co., 1980. Distributed by United Ostomy Association.

Nessim and Ellis, *Cancervive: The Challenge of Life after Cancer*, Houghton Mifflin Co., New York, 1991.

Pinckney and Swenson, *New Image for Women*, Acropolis Books Ltd., Washington D.C., 1984.

Siegel, *Love, Medicine and Miracles*, Harper and Row, New York, 1986.

Siegel, *Peace, Love, and Healing*, Harper and Row, New York, 1989.

Simonton, Matthews-Simonton, and Crieghton, *Getting Well Again*, Bantam Books, New York, 1978.

Winter, *A Consumer's Dictionary of Cosmetic Ingredients*, Crown, New York, 1984.

Zeman, *Clinical Nutrition and Dietetics,* The Collamore Press, Lexington, Massachusetts, 1983.

PAMPHLETS

American Cancer Society Patient Education Booklet. Available through local chapters.

F.D.A. Consumer, Department of Health and Human Services, Public Health Service, Food and Drug Administration, Office of Public Affairs, 5600 Fisher Lane, Rockville, Maryland, 20857.

The Leukemia Society Patient Education Booklets. Available at local chapters or by calling 1-800-955-4LSA.

National Cancer Institute Patient Education Booklets. Call the Cancer Information Service, 1-800-4-CANCER for free educational booklets on a variety of subjects.

Nutrition: A Helpful Ally in Cancer Therapy, Ross Laboratories, Division of Medical Nutritionals, Columbus, OH 43216.

U.S. Department of Health and Human Services, *Chemotherapy and You*, National Cancer Institute, Bethesda, Maryland.

When Eating Right is a Jungle, The Doyle Pharmaceutical Co., 5320 West 23rd St., Minneapolis, MN 55416.

HAIR ALTERNATIVES

Crowning Touch
Nisus Concepts, Inc.
P.O. Box 143
Glen Haven, CO 80532
(303) 586-9204

Specializes in fashion headwear for the woman experiencing hair loss. Call or write for brochure.

Designs for Comfort, Inc.
P.O. Box 8229
Northfield, IL 60093
(800) 443-9226
Illinois residents: (708) 446-9190
FAX: (708) 446-9224

Designs for Comfort has developed a combination cap and hairpiece called the "Headliner". It is a comfortable and an attractive alternative to wigs. The "Headliner" is available in a variety of colors and fabrics. This product may be reimbursed by individual insurance companies as a hair prosthesis. Brochure available. Call or write for information regarding local retailers.

Jeffery Paul
Hair Replacement and Cosmetic
Reconstruction Specialists
20595 Lorain Road
Fairview Park, Ohio 44126
(216) 333-8939

Jeffery Paul Hair Replacement and Cosmetic Reconstruction Center was established to help meet the needs of individuals visibly scarred by disease, injury, or trauma. Services provided include hair replacement for partial or complete hair loss and cosmetic camouflage. Call for an appointment.

The Judy Stewart Collection
P.O. Box 4262
Bellingham, WA 98277
(206) 676-9458

Fashion headwraps and turbans designed to fit the special needs of women and children experiencing hair loss due to cancer therapy. Call or write for brochure.

Just in Time
P.O. Box 27693
Philadelphia, PA 19118
(215) 247-8777

Headwear designed specifically for women experiencing hair loss. All selections are reversible, made of 100% cotton, and are hand washable. Just in Time also makes a scarf pad, worn under scarves or turbans gives the illusion of a full head of hair tucked underneath.

Look Yourself Corporation
20595 Lorain Avenue
Fairview Park, Ohio 44126
(216) 333-8939

The Look Yourself Corporation is the business of educating the public and professionals about hair loss. Seminars are offered throughout the United States and Canada. Their video "A Patient's Guide to Hair Replacement Options" is available for loan to patients, and comes with a complimentary 8-page illustrated book. Call or write for information.

P.K. Walsh
1842 Beacon Street
Brookline, MA 02146
(617) 232-4521

Provides a large selection of hair alternatives for women, men, and children experiencing medical and genetic hair loss. P.K. Walsh also offers private fitting rooms, free initial consultations, and makeup and styling assistance. Call for an appointment.

Peggy Knight International
32 Ross Common, Box 1642
Ross, California 94957-1642
(415) 461-4395
(800) 333-8018
FAX (415) 461-4399

Specializes in synthetic and human hair wigs
for individuals experiencing total or partial
hair loss. Hair consultants are available
nationwide. The Peggy Knight Center for
Women, locations in Northern California,
provide services and products to help women
with their physical appearance during cancer
treatments including: hairpieces, turbans,
scarves, breast forms, and makeup
consultation. Brochure available. Call or
write for information.

Professional Hairgoods
302 West 238 Street
Riverdale, New York 10463
(212) 884-6024
FAX (212) 601-1932

Professional Hairgoods sells all styles of
human and synthetic wigs for men, women,
and children. Providing wigs for every taste
and every budget, this business is particularly
sensitive to the needs of the person
experiencing hair loss from cancer therapy.
Consultants available nationwide. Mail order
service. Call or write for information.

Special Treatment
338 North Orange Drive
Los Angeles, CA 90036
(213) 934-1760

Linda Secher, owner and founder, feels she is
an extension of home care. Servicing most of
Southern California, she provides on-site
consultations, meeting patients at the location
of their choice. She provides a full range
of hair alternatives for women, men, and
children experiencing hair loss from cancer
therapies.

Styl-Rama, Inc.
Hair Replacement and Cosmetic
Rehabilitation Center
Courtside Square
150 Allendale Road
King of Prussia, Pennsylvania 19406
(215) 337-2696

A full-service salon specializing in traumatic
hair loss. Complete product line of hair loss
options for women, men, and children. Private
consultation suites. Call for an appointment.

"Top Secret"
1015 3rd Street Promenade, Suite 18
Santa Monica, CA 90401
(310) 393-7433

Full service custom made wig studio
specializing in the needs of women, men, and
children following chemotherapy. Call for an
appointment.

HAIR LOSS REFERRAL SOURCES

The following organizations can help you find
a local appearance consultant who specializes
in hair loss from cancer therapy.

Hair Loss Council
100 Independence Place, Suite 207
Tyler, TX 75703
(903) 561-1107
(800) 274-8717

National Alopecia Areata Foundation
714 C. Street, Suite 202
San Rafael, CA 94901
(415) 456-4644

FASHION AND BEAUTY SUPPLY

Adam's Specialty Shop
18545 Roscoe Boulevard
Northridge, California 91324
(818) 993-8556

Service is the number one priority at Adam's Specialty Shop. There is an extensive selection of breast forms, bras, lingerie, post-mastectomy accessories, swim wear, and sportswear. The staff is friendly and knowledgeable about post-mastectomy care and insurance reimbursement issues. All consultations are done in large private suites. An on-site seamstress will customize any garment to meet the customer's special needs. Lymphedema care is also provided. Call for an appointment.

Alra Radiation Therapy Lotion
Alra Research Laboratories
711 South Main Street
Burbank, CA 91506
(800) 832-8311

Alra means "all radiation" and was specifically formulated with the consultation of a radiation oncologist to counteract and relieve those special skin problems (dryness and scaling) associated with radiation therapy. It is non-greasy, light on the skin, and free of fragrance and alcohol. Call or write for a brochure.

Hair by Chemo
Box 223
Wauzeka, Wisconsin 53826
1-800-729-9713

A brother and sister team, both cancer survivors, developed this line of fashion wear. "Hair by Chemo, Not by Choice" is the emblem of courage (and humor) that is proudly displayed on baseball caps, t-shirts, and sweatshirts. Call for information.

Johanna's of Albany, Ltd.
199 New Scotland Avenue
Albany, NY 12208
(518) 482-4178

"On call to mend esteem," Johanna's of Albany provides services and products aimed at those individuals of all ages with an altered body image due to cancer therapy. Services include hair loss alternatives, post-mastectomy care, ostomy care, mobile out-reach programs, and cancer awareness programs. Mail order catalog and a variety of patient audio-visual available. Call or write for information.

Mary Catherine's
4107 N.E. Tillamook St.
Portland, Oregon 97212
1-800-654-9957 (Oregon only)
1-800-843-3215 (outside Oregon)

A complete intimate apparel boutique for women after breast surgery. Write for their mail order catalog, it provides a large selection of bras, prostheses, and swim wear.

Michael Maron's Makeover Magic
Professional Undermakeup System
P.O. Box 1335
Hampton Bays, NY 11946
(800) 248-2211

The Professional Undermakeup System can conceal almost any skin imperfections such as post-surgical scars and changes in skin pigmentation. Step-by-step illustrated brochure and how-to video included. Call for information.

149

Style n' Motion
8805 Solon Road, Suite G1
Houston, TX 77064
1-800-524-6688
Texas residents, (713) 894-6088

Style n' Motion gives adults and children a
way to liven up and personalize their
wheelchairs with colorful upholstery and
accessories. Sixteen different chair styles are
available, as well as over 20 different colors
and designs. Call or write for a full color
brochure.

SUPPORT ORGANIZATIONS

American Cancer Society
3340 Peachtree Road, NE
Atlanta, Georgia 30026
1-800-ACS-2345

The American Cancer Society is a volunteer
organization that provides information,
support, and financial resources to cancer
patients, their families, the community, and
health care professionals. In addition, there
are many separate programs geared to the
special situations unique to specific types of
cancers, such as Reach to Recovery for
women with mastectomies. The American
Cancer Society has divisions in all major
cities in the United States. For more
information about an office near you
contact the national office.

Burger King Cancer Caring Center
4117 Liberty Avenue
Pittsburgh, PA 15224
(412) 622-1212

Cancer Lifeline
500 Lowman Building
107 Cherry Street
Seattle, WA 98104
(206) 461-4542 (Seattle)
(800) 255-5505 (Washington State only)

Cancer Lifeline provides emotional support
and resources for cancer patients, their
families, and friends. Services are provided
through a state-wide, 24 hour toll-free phone
number, family meetings, and community
education.

Corporate Angel Network, Inc.
Westchester County Airport, Building 1
White Plains, NY 10604
(914) 328-1313

A service which provides free rides on
corporate airplanes for specialized cancer
treatments.

**Encore - (Encouragement, Normalcy,
Counseling, Opportunity, Reaching Out,
Energies Revived)**
YWCA - National Office
126 Broadway
New York, NY 10003

Provides support for post-operative breast
cancer patients. Encore meetings include
exercise and discussion sessions.

Hats, Hair, and Huggybears
199 New Scotland Avenue
Albany, New York 12208
(518) 482-4178

Hats, Hair, and Huggybears is a non-profit
foundation that provides education, support,
and assistance to children, adolescents, and

teens who suffer hair loss as a consequence of cancer therapy.

Look Good, Feel Better
The C.T.F.A. Foundation
The Cosmetic, Toiletry and Fragrance Association
1110 Vermont Ave. NW, Suite 800
Washington D.C. 20005
(202) 331-1770
(800) 395-LOOK

Look Good, Feel Better is a joint nationwide public service program between the C.T.F.A. and the American Cancer Society designed to assist the person recovering from cancer to enhance their quality of life through personal appearance and body image. The focus of the program is makeup and skin care issues; however, there are regional differences in how the program is implemented. Contact your local American Cancer Society for additional information.

National Cancer Institute
1-800-4-CANCER
CancerFax: (301) 402-5874

Accurate, personalized answers to your cancer-related questions are only a phone call away. The Cancer Information Service is a nationwide toll-free telephone program, sponsored by the National Cancer Institute, providing information on all aspects of cancer prevention, detection, diagnosis, and treatment. Spanish-speaking staff members are available to callers from the following areas (daytime hours only): California, Florida, Georgia, Illinois, Northern New Jersey, New York City, and Texas. CancerFax

is the newest patient information resource sponsored by the N.C.I. Simply dial 1-301-402-5874 on your facsimile machine and listen to the instructions.

The National Coalition for
Cancer Survivorship
1010 Wayne Avenue, Suite 300
Silverspring, Maryland 20910
(301) 585-2616

The N.C.C.S. was established to facilitate communication between people affected by cancer survivorship issues (i.e., insurance, job discrimination...). Call the national headquarters for information on local chapters, membership, and conventions.

The National Lymphatic and
Venous Foundation, Inc.
P.O. Box 242
Cambridge, MA 02141

The National Lymphatic and Venous Foundation is a non-profit organization dedicated to helping all individuals who are affected by chronic lymphedema and venous diseases. Newsletter available. Write for information.

United Ostomy Association - National
Office
36 Executive Park, Suite 120
Irvine, CA 92714
(714) 660-8624

The United Ostomy Association is dedicated to helping people with ostomies return to normal living. Provides support services and education in its chapters nationwide.

151

The Wellness Community
Main Office
1235 5th St.
Santa Monica, CA 90401
(310) 393-1415

The Wellness Community is a model,
non-profit program for people with cancer. It
is supported by individuals and organizations
who believe that people with cancer who
participate in their own recovery will
substantially improve the quality of their lives
and may enhance the probability of recovery.
A variety of educational and support programs
are provided.

Y-Me Breast Cancer Support Program, Inc.
18220 Harwood
Homewood, IL 60430
(312) 799-8338
Hotline: (800) 221-2141
Chicago area: (312) 799-8228

Y-Me is a not-for-profit organization that
provides information, hotline counseling,
educational programs, and self-help meetings
for breast cancer patients, their families,
and friends.

PERSONAL RESOURCES

List names and phone numbers.

Doctor _____

Hospital _____

Pharmacy _____

Local American Cancer Society

_____

Support Organizations

_____

_____

_____

Wigs

_____

_____

_____

Headwraps

_____

_____

_____

Mail Order

_____

_____

_____

Makeup Supplies

_____

_____

_____

Sunscreen

_____

_____

_____

Skin Care Products

_____

_____

_____

Other

_____

_____

_____

Index

C

157

Notes

Notes

Notes

Notes

ABOUT THE AUTHORS

Diane Doan Noyes is a sales representative for Laurel Burch, Inc. For over a decade she has been involved in the sales and marketing of women's fashions and accessories. Recognized by her peers as a role model, she has received several awards acknowledging her accomplishments, including the Susan B. Komen award for outstanding work with cancer patients and *Cosmopolitan* magazine's Career Woman of the Month. Her personal experience with the side effects of chemotherapy inspired her to launch a program aimed at educating the fashion and cosmetic industry about the cosmetic solutions for the side effects of cancer therapy. She is on the founding board of the National Coalition of Cancer Survivorship, Seattle chapter. She lives in Seattle with her husband.

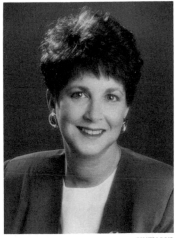

YUEN LUI

Peggy Mellody is a registered nurse specializing in oncology. As a consultant, writer, and lecturer she has earned a reputation as an active and respected cancer authority. She is the author of numerous publications for cancer patients, their families, and medical and nursing staff. Author of *The Los Angeles Food Guide*, *Sweet Celebrations*, and co-author of *Cobblers, Crumbles, and Crisps*, and *In the Chips: The Complete Chocolate Chip Cookbook*, she has successfully combined a career in nursing and an interest in the culinary arts. While continuing to write, she works as an alternate site oncology infusion specialist. She currently lives in Los Angeles with her husband.

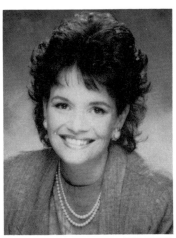

E.K. WALLER

171

Order Form ▬▬▬▬▬▬

Please send me additional copies of Beauty & Cancer.

Name: _____

Company: _____

Address: _____

City/State/Zip: _____

Telephone: _____

Please send _____ copy(ies) @ $12.95 $_____

Shipping and Handling @ $2.00 each $_____

Total $_____

Please make check payable to: Taylor Publishing Company
Attention: Trade Books
1550 West Mockingbird Lane
Dallas, Texas 75235

1-800-275-8188 (for credit card orders only)